D1801446

SECOND EDITION

THE BIG
BOOK OF
Care
Plans

Best Practices for Interdisciplinary
Assessments and Care Planning

Debbie Ohl, RN, NHA, M.Msc.

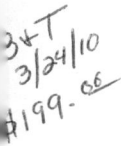

HCPro

The Big Book of Care Plans: Best Practices for Interdisciplinary Assessments and Care Planning, Second Edition is published by HCPro, Inc.

Copyright © 2009, 2006 HCPro, Inc.

All rights reserved. Printed in the United States of America.   5   4   3   2   1

ISBN: 978-1-60146-324-1

HCPro, Inc., provides information resources for the healthcare industry.

HCPro, Inc., is not affiliated in any way with The Joint Commission, which owns the JCAHO and Joint Commission trademarks.

Debbie Ohl, RN, NHA, M.Msc., Author
Adrienne Trivers, Managing Editor
Elizabeth Petersen, Executive Editor
Emily Sheahan, Group Publisher
Shane Katz, Cover Designer
Mike Mirabello, Senior Graphic Artist

Audrey Doyle, Copyeditor
Alison Forman, Proofreader
Darren Kelly, Books Production Supervisor
Susan Darbyshire, Art Director
Jean St. Pierre, Director of Operations

Advice given is general. Readers should consult professional counsel for specific legal, ethical, or clinical questions.

Arrangements can be made for quantity discounts. For more information, contact:

HCPro, Inc.
P.O. Box 1168
Marblehead, MA 01945
Telephone: 800/650-6787 or 781/639-1872
Fax: 781/639-2982
E-mail: *customerservice@hcpro.com*

Visit HCPro at its World Wide Web sites:
www.hcpro.com and *www.hcmarketplace.com*

Contents

About the Author

Debbie Ohl, RN, NHA, M.Msc.

Debbie Ohl, RN, NHA, M.Msc., is the owner and senior consultant of Ohl & Associates, a long-term care education, resource, and consulting company based in Cincinnati. Ms. Ohl is a veteran consultant to long-term care providers including nursing facilities and hospitals throughout the nation. Ms. Ohl is considered to be unsurpassed in her understanding of and expertise in virtually all clinical and regulatory areas affecting long-term care nursing facilities.

Author of more than a dozen books on subjects related to nursing home administration and long-term care, Ms. Ohl is a sought-after speaker and seminar facilitator. Ms. Ohl founded Ohl & Associates in 1980 in response to increasing demands and growing regulatory complexities. Her most recent accomplishment is the creation of care planning software that parallels *The Big Book of Care Plans*. Ms. Ohl believes that the process and outcome of care planning are the foundation for creating excellence in care.

The Practice of Care Planning

Care Plans, Then and Now

Since the words "where's the care plan" were first uttered by a state surveyor in the mid-1970s, a progressive blueprint has emerged. It's said that it takes 10 years to change a paradigm or pattern. Understanding the advances in care plan substance and content makes it easier to recognize what is and is not appropriate for care planning in the twenty-first century.

1970s care plans

A new idea in the mid-1970s, care plans were the latest expectations of regulators and emphasized the idea of having a plan for each resident. Substance and content were low priorities. Instead, the focus was on establishing the habit of creating a care plan.

Toward the end of the 1970s, expectations were raised. Surveyors told us that every diagnosis must be addressed (the birth of the medical model care plan) and every discipline must create a care plan for each resident (the multidisciplinary approach). Each discipline looked at the nursing care plan and picked a part to address. Falling short of this mandate meant a deficiency.

Shortly following these edicts, we were told that every medication must be addressed on the care plan. Before you knew it, plans were as thick as encyclopedias, though no one except surveyors ever looked at them. Twenty-page care plans were the norm. Paper compliance was the name of the game.

1980s care plans

As the 1980s emerged, the care plan habit was falling into place, though entries were not timely, goals weren't measurable, reasonable, or appropriate, functional problems were infrequently addressed, and care plans were written after the fact in an attempt to avoid deficiencies.

During this period, the idea of measurable goals came to the forefront. Surveyors advised, "Use numbers." So, often like sheep to the slaughter, we began to make sure our goals were able to be measured, though what they were actually measuring in the way of outcomes was up for grabs (e.g., "Resident will be able to walk 10 feet." And this will do what for the resident?). Nonetheless, we were learning the concept.

In addition to measurable goals, surveyors also started to pay attention to interventions: Were they present? Did they identify the responsible discipline? Were they specific? The tone of regulator wants placed impossible demands on nursing facilities, but nursing facilities were conditioned to do what they were told. Because the interventions were not realistic, this invariably led to more deficiencies. For example: "TIAN (toilet in advance of need) every two hours. Presented as 'You need to do this if any resident is incontinent of urine.' " That was not written in the regulations or the interpretive guidelines, but for an industry not paying proper attention to the problem of incontinence, it got our attention. And again, like sheep to the slaughter, we wrote these care plans and then received deficiencies because this rigid schedule, which was inappropriate for most residents, could not possibly be followed. Once the habit was established, improvement in assessing and managing incontinence ultimately came about.

Emphasis in the 1980s was on the paper, step one in conditioning now complete. The Omnibus Budget Reconciliation Act came along in 1987. It was the first major revision of federal standards for nursing home care since the 1965 creation of both Medicare and Medicaid. Long-term care facilities participating in Medicare or Medicaid were to provide services to insure that each resident could "attain and maintain her highest practicable physical, mental, and psycho-social well-being." and it was time for another milestone: The concept of resident-centered care was born.

1990s care plans

Behavior problems and restraints were major issues in the early 1990s. Regulatory mandates demanded care plans for use of restraints with strict guidelines. This called for validating and rationalizing the need for use, and linked the clinical assessment process to the care plan. Until this point, plans were based on resident symptoms with the emphasis on controlling the symptom, not necessarily using the clinical process to determine cause and contributors for the symptoms. Symptom-based care plans are medical model care plans. In the 1990s, the concept of holistic care was emerging. Holistic care is a synonym for comprehensive care, which is based on total care of the resident. Holistic healthcare considers the physical, emotional, social, economic, and spiritual needs of the person. With the shift from the medical model to the holistic care model, the individual resident became more than a diagnosis and symptoms. The seed for resident-centered care plans and the use of clinical assessment in developing care plans was beginning to grow, facilitated by the resident assessment instrument.

In addition, care conferences were looked at more closely. Facilities were beginning to shift from a paper-shuffling approach to a discussion of resident status with a perfunctory review of the care plan. Achievement of stated goals was looked at more closely. Extended goal dates with no progress or rationale came under scrutiny. Resident and family participation at the care conference was beginning to come about.

Care teams no longer called themselves *multidisciplinary*, but rather *interdisciplinary*, meaning they worked together to address resident needs. Facilities struggled greatly with this; some still do. The philosophical ideal was in place, but the old medical model for care plan development did not lend itself well to the interdisciplinary model. The idea was there, but in reality the practice was lacking. Nonetheless, care plans were moving toward a more holistic model, and functional status of the resident was being included. Care plans continued to be lengthy, done by a few and occasionally looked at by the floor staff.

Care plans of the twenty-first century

Today, computerized care plans are being used to a degree, but they lack personalization, and tailoring to individual needs proves challenging. The nurses on the unit are just beginning to become involved in the process as an expected action. Timely care plan entries and knowledge of content is a more familiar practice on healthcare units. Surveyors focus on resident-based care plan goals and interventions; staff members are expected to know these. The outcomes are now geared toward maintenance and enhancement of functional status and quality of life.

The care planning process has moved from paper to practice. The Centers for Medicare & Medicaid Services' (CMS) interpretative guidelines have become more defined. Quality of care is an expected outcome in facilities across the country. Quality of life has become the centerpiece of care planning. More resident participation and involvement is expected, along with new ways to ensure this, even among the cognitively challenged. Another major shift in thinking for nursing facilities is required.

The new challenge is to create relevant, focused, personalized care plans that reflect who the person is, documenting and doing what the person wants, in his or her way. To improve our thinking and rationale, interpretive guidelines are now underscoring the importance of documenting rationale. No rationale for action means a deficiency will be coming your way. This is particularly evident in areas that are potentially high risk for negative resident outcomes. A prime example is the interpretive guidelines unnecessary medication criteria that demands very specific documentation to validate use of medications. Typically, regulators pick one area to hit hard; the new habit gets established, and like a pebble in a pond the habit spreads to other areas.

Personalized care plans humanize the resident. They support us in seeing the individual as a person with a life story, a person who has history and who deserves the utmost respect and consideration. The care plan is the tool that will begin to put this principle into action. It has taken several decades to bring us to this point.

New ideas are being discussed as to the best methodology to bring this high-minded ideal into daily practice. Person-centered care plans tackle this concept from a subjective perspective: If this were me, given my lifetime values, preferences, and history, what would I want? Once you experience this shift, you will have moved from resident-centered care to person-centered care.

Twentieth-century objective

Resident-centered care

Resident-centered care is driven by quality of care and is non-personalized. You are meeting the particular care needs, but the approach is more task-oriented and structured to the facility.

Twenty-first-century objective

Person-centered care

Person-centered care is driven by quality of life as the resident defines it. You are caring for this particular human being according to his or her unique habits and preferences. The approach is more person-driven.

The care plan is the mechanism to insure personalized and meaningful care, insuring that the resident receives the highest quality of care and services to maintain and enhance his or her physical, mental, and psychosocial well being. *The Big Book of Care Plans* has been designed to promote this process and provide the necessary tools to achieve these goals.

Medications and Care Planning

Given the heavy emphasis on medication use, when you are thinking about care planning you should consider the risk of the medication being used. If it is a high-risk medication such as a psychoactive medication, consider a separate care plan that addresses the rationale for medication use, as well as the resident's current baseline and expected outcome, a time table for administration and risk factors to which you should be alerted.

Although side effects can materialize at any time, review of literature indicates that the window is typically three days to 12 weeks. A good rule of thumb is to consider medications started, stopped, or changed in the past 30 days as a possible cause or contributor to a status change or worsening conditioning.

Keep in mind that a medication can be a problem, need, or risk requiring a care plan in and of itself, or that the medication can be an intervention in and of itself. The challenge is to decide which position it holds on the plan: a problem/need or an intervention.

Medication use is a key component in the clinical process. The Federal Medication Guidelines are designed to ensure that use of medications is of value and is necessary, and places significant emphasis on preventing and recognizing adverse drug reactions.

Consequently, surveyors expect to see rationale for use, parameters for monitoring, prompt recognition and evaluation of new onset problems and worsening conditions, and consideration for reducing and discontinuing medication as appropriate. Failure to comply with the guidelines can result in an unnecessary drug citation. Assessment, care plan development, implementation, and monitoring are the supporting foundation for compliance.

Unnecessary Medication	
Excessive doses	Given at one time or over a period of time
Excessive duration	Longer than required or needed
Without adequate monitoring	System not in place; missed changes in status indicating need for action
Without adequate indications for use	Failure to establish rationale for use
Presence of adverse consequences indicating dose should be reduced or discontinued	Failure to recognize change and/or take action as indicated or needed

Non-compliance also creates the following potential deficiencies:

- Unnecessary drug use

- Antipsychotic drug use

- Medication errors

- Drug regimen review

- Comprehensive assessment

- Care planning

- Professional standards of practice

To prevent these interrelationships consider the following:

- Do the target symptoms warrant medications?

- Are non-pharmacological interventions in place and relevant?

- Is medication appropriate for managing the symptoms or condition?

- Do the intended or actual benefits justify the risk of use?

- Is a system in place to ensure that these processes are adhered to?

Surveyor looks for:	Facility Actions MUST ESTABLISH BASELINE
Indications/reasons for use	Assessment and rationale for use documented
Dose and effectiveness	Dose range, expected outcome, and timeline
Monitoring	Drug regimen review, timely response to irregularities
Duplication of drug therapy (same class, similar side effects)	Drug regimen review, timely response to irregularities
Presence of adverse drug events (predictable verses unpredictable)	Recognition: requires knowledge of baseline, known drug side effects
Weight history of note	Triggers: gain, loss, anorexia, dysphagia
Hydration/intake of note	Triggers: change in hydration, fluid, electrolyte balance

There are five reasons for using medication. Consider these as you assess and plan care:

1. Cure an acute illness

2. Arrest or slow the disease process

3. Decrease or eliminate symptoms

4. Prevent a disease or symptom

5. Therapeutic or enabling for a resident with chronic mental or physical problems

The Unnecessary Drugs Guidelines encompass all medications given. Psychoactive and Beers Criteria medications are the highest risk and will require care planning. To assist in effective care planning, review the questions and strategies in these areas.

Assessment Questions Regarding Psychoactive Medications and Behavior

- What is the behavior? How long does it last?

- Is the behavior a threat, distressing, or harmful to the resident or others?

- Are psychoactive medications used?

- Is the behavior creating care resistance, or is the care creating the behavior problem?

© 2009 HCPro, Inc.

- What are the potential causes or contributors to the behavior problem?

- Can the behavior be easily altered? If not, why not?

- Has the use of medication been considered?

- Have you evaluated the triggered resident assessment protocols and triggered quality indicators?

- Are supporting criteria for the drug category being used?

Treatment Principles for Behavior Management

- Rule out and/or stabilize medical problems

- Check critical lab work

- Create a list of behavior disturbances that need to be improved

- Augment therapy if needed

- Set realistic goals

- Establish a routine for the cognitively impaired

- Provide physical clues for the cognitively impaired

- Talk before touching

- Use one-step commands for the cognitively impaired

- Allow adequate time for medication trial

- Specify and quantify improvement

Critical Questions When Using Behavior and Psychoactive Medication

- What are the symptoms?

- What is the frequency?

- What is the ease of alterability?

If easily altered:

- Is the resident receiving psychoactive meds?

- How long?

- Are side effects present?

- Is a reduction program needed or underway?

If not easily altered:

- Have physical causes been ruled out?

- Might drug interactions be creating the problem? How do you know?

- Is the resident receiving psych meds? How long? Has the resident's behavior improved? If not, why not? What do you plan to do now?

Critical Questions When Using Depression and Psychoactive Medication

- What are the symptoms?

- If you don't think these symptoms are mood-related, why?

- How have you come to this decision?

- How pervasive are the symptoms?

- How serious are the symptoms?

- How easily altered are the symptoms?

- Are psychoactive, antianxiety, or hypnotics therapies in use?

If the resident is easily altered and receiving an antidepressant is the resident a candidate for reduction?

If the resident is *not* easily altered and is receiving an antidepressant how long has the resident been receiving the medication?

If the resident is *not* easily altered and is *not* receiving antidepressant is the resident a candidate for receiving an antidepressant?

Beers Criteria

Beers Criteria is a guideline that looks specifically at potentially inappropriate medications in the *over elderly* as 65 population. The Beers List includes medications with high-risk side effects outweighing any benefit the medication may have at any dose, for any indication, and medications to be used with caution at certain doses and for specific indications. The following med classes are frequently used in long-term care. Refer to the complete Beers List easily available via an Internet search.

- **Anticholinergic medications:** tricyclic antidepressants; antihistamines; antispasmodics and muscle relaxants. Adverse effects: urinary retention; constipation; confusion; delirium; behavior changes; exacerbation of dementia

- **Antianxiety/sedative agents:** select short-acting agents; lowest possible dose; shortest possible time; evaluate need for therapy frequently

- **Antipsychotics:** use least-sedating agents; minimal anticholinergic effects

- **Antidepressants:** use least-sedating agents; minimal cardiotoxicity; minimal anticholinergic side effects

- **Antihypertensives:** all

Pain and Care Planning

Pain has the potential to affect both quality of care and quality of life. Pain management is a crucial component in care planning and regulatory compliance. You can improve an effective care plan for managing pain with some basic information on the subject of pain.

What is pain?

Pain is whatever the person says it is. Pain is an unpleasant sensory or emotional experience that is primarily associated with tissue damage or described in terms of tissue damage, or both. Pain is a complex perception that takes place only at higher levels of the central nervous system.

What is quality of life?

Quality of life is a manner or way of existing. Quality of life focuses on the person, not the resident. All of the surveyor protocols reflect this perspective.

What is quality of care?

Quality of care is the degree of excellence in care provided. Most nursing home residents are at risk of physical decline; most have multiple chronic illnesses and a variety of factors that severely impact self-sufficiency. Activities of daily living (ADLs) decline and other negative clinical outcomes prompt investigation of pain presence and management as a modifiable root cause or outcome. These factors, coupled with inadequate pain management, have prompted CMS to investigate how care planning strives to impact the quality of a resident's life.

What to Consider When Care Planning

Pain behaviors

Pain behaviors are certain actions that a patient may present with that are either verbal or non-verbal, such as guarding, restriction of movement, rubbing of the affected area, grimacing, or sighing. In short, pain behaviors can include the following:

- Non-verbal sounds

- Facial expressions

- Bracing, guarding, rubbing, or massaging a body part

- Restlessness, agitation, combativeness, fidgeting, pacing, or withdrawal

- Changes in mental status

- Changes in interpersonal interactions

Pain threshold

Pain threshold is the least experience of pain that a patient can recognize.

Pain tolerance level

Pain tolerance level is the greatest level of pain that a patient is prepared to tolerate.

Palliative

Palliative refers to a treatment, which can be surgical or pharmacological, that attempts to relieve or alleviate pain, but without the goal of curing. Palliative care can be provided through medical intervention, or it can be pharmaceutical or surgical in nature, and is performed with the goal of managing untoward symptoms and improving quality of life, rather than altering or curing a disease.

Breakthrough pain

The following symptoms characterize breakthrough pain:

- A sudden flare-up that "breaks through" the pain medication taken for a persistent pain

- A typical episode may peak in as little as three minutes and last 30 minutes

- Up to 85% of people with persistent pain also experience breakthrough pain

- Breakthrough pain is different from persistent pain and requires different treatment

Assessment Questions for Personalized Care Planning and Pain

- Where does it hurt? Does the pain move from one place to another?

- Do you have more than one spot where it hurts? When does the pain happen?

- How long does it last? Does the pain come and go? Or is it there all the time?

- Is this pain new? Have you ever had this pain before? When does it begin? When does it end?

- Does the pain keep you from doing all that you want to do?

- Does the pain interrupt your sleep? Does it change your mood? Affect your appetite?

- What makes the pain better? What makes it worse? What have you tried to relieve the pain?

- How long does the medicine take to work? How long does relief last? Does all of the pain go away after you take the medicine? Does the pain return before the next dose is due?

Pain Risk Factors Worksheet

The more factors present, the higher the probability that pain is present.

- Cognitive impairment
- 85 years of age or older
- Female
- Pain med given PRN

- Minority
- Behavior problems
- Mood problems
- Med given routinely

- Psychoactive med use
- Diagnosis can cause pain
- Pain med ordered
- Other pain management in place

Consider creating protocols for types of pain to lessen the care planning burden.

- For each type of pain include the specific medical interventions and non-medical interventions, including service providers and/or the particular discipline:

  1. Acute pain
     – Mild
     – Moderate
     – Severe

  2. Persistent/chronic pain
     – Mild
     – Moderate
     – Severe

  3. Severe/excruciating pain
     – Occasional
     – Intermittent
     – Constant

Care Plan Development with Pain As the Root Problem

Components of Pain Care Plan: Analgesia, Quality of Life, Ability to Function

PROBLEM/NEED/STRENGTH	GOAL(S) What does the resident want?	REVIEW Date	APPROACHES/ INTERVENTIONS	RESPONSIBLE DISCIPLINE
Issue: Why pain **Description** of pain: type, source, location, intensity **Resulting** in/creating/impacting: effect on functional status PMS/E: Physical, mental, social, emotional **Risks/complication:** *(resulting from pain and medication used)* **Resident strengths:**	**Resolve and eliminate** the issue if possible **Pain relief/control** **Quality of life:** - What can you make better? - What is the best you can expect?		**Medication plan** Who can do: What When Where How often	

ILLUSTRATION

Problem/Need/Want	Goal(s)
Severe pain secondary to back injury, **resulting in** escalation of chronic depression and anxiety, resulting in risk for: P: Reduced mobility, urinary incontinence, falls and pressure ulcers, dehydration, and weight loss M: Confusion, disorientation S/E: Escalation in chronic depression and anxiety, creating risk for reduced decision-making and poor motivation to participate in recovery Strengths: Alert, oriented, capable of making decisions	Pain will be minimized/relieved as evidenced by resident statement of same and desire to be out of room for dinner Will continue to make decisions about care Mobility will not be compromised as evidenced by continuing to walk with assist of cane and coming to dining room for dinner Will remain continent of urine Will be without falls and skin will remain intact Will be adequately hydrated as evidenced by frequent, clear urination Weight will remain within 1 to 2 lbs of 125 lbs. Will remain alert and oriented as evidenced by conversation of current events Will actively participate in recovery via attending therapy and restorative nursing activities

To capture the credit certain pieces of documentation must be in place:

Assessment	MDS, triggered RAP, clinical assessment as indicated
Care Plan	• Defined functional problem • Measurable goal(s) and time frames • Intervention including specific approaches • Frequency of service • Time of service • Service provider
Delivery Records	Reflect provision of service, service provider, and time spent
Periodic Progress Notes	Not defined by rule. Therefore, the facility sets the standard for frequency of entries. Keep in mind that these are *not* paper programs, but rather programs with a purpose. Therefore, documentation is a tool to reflect and prompt needed actions to ensure the best results. **Recommended frequency:** On initiation, and daily x 1 week, then weekly x 4, then monthly, until the team feels quarterly notes are adequate.* ** Generally after the resident and staff members have firmly established the activity as routine performance and the status is very stable.*

Restorative Nursing Care Planning

Restorative Care Planning

Rehabilitative and restorative care in the geriatric setting is a philosophical approach that recognizes diagnosis and age as poor predictors of functional ability. Interventions in the long-term care setting are directed toward enhanced performance.

Rehabilitative potential is the ability of the resident to reach goals, and is a judgment of the probable course and outcomes of the disease or condition. The satisfaction of the resident is a primary benchmark for determining the success or failure of a restorative program. Improving the quality of life from the perspective of the individual rather than what the therapist or nurse considers as improvement is a critical component of rehab and restorative programs.

Prognosis is the likelihood of maintaining independent or improved function. In the nursing facility, maintenance of achieved functional status has been a challenge. Status declines once formal therapy or restorative nursing is discontinued—a situation which occurs too frequently in the healthcare setting.

The regulatory environment, enhanced assessment tools such as the Minimum Data Set (MDS) and resident assessment protocols (RAPs), and the use of quality indicators, coupled with an industry of professionals with growing competency, have all come together to spearhead true improvements of a continuous nature in the nursing facility. The focus on care provided, outcomes, functional status, and quality of life demands an aggressive approach to maintenance and enhancement of resident status.

Regardless of what form or format you use for assessment and care planning, if you do not use the information on the forms you are merely making a paper-compliant attempt to deal with regulatory requirements. It is essential that the paper and corresponding documentation be the means to the end (i.e., that it positively affects resident outcomes).

The objective of the documentation tools in this manual is to provide clinical staff members with a structured format for paying prompt attention to items they need to consider when assessing residents and developing and implementing their care plans.

To be effective the documentation tools *must be individualized.* You can accomplish this by checking the pertinent information in each section and adding any additional information to further tailor each plan to each individual.

Do not use these forms if you are unwilling or unable to ensure that they are individualized and used to facilitate the assessment and care planning processes.

Please note: *The user assumes all responsibility for use of the materials in this manual. The user is strongly cautioned to review regulatory and reimbursement requirements to ensure compliance, as regulations and interpretations vary and change over time.*

Restorative Nursing Care Plan Program

Goal specifics

- To emphasize ability and deemphasize disability; that is, to focus on what is left and not on what is missing

- To promote self-care responsibility

- To foster independence

- To reinforce skills learned in formal therapy

- To teach functional adaptation when complete recovery is not possible

 The Big Book of Care Plans, Second Edition

Program requirements: MDS 2.0, Item P3

1. Measurable objectives and interventions must be documented in the care plan and in the clinical record.

2. Evidence of periodic evaluation by a licensed nurse is necessary.

3. Nurse assistants/aides must be trained in the techniques that promote resident involvement in the activity.

4. These activities must be carried out *or* supervised by members of the nursing staff.

Sometimes under licensed nurse supervision, other staff members and volunteers may be assigned to work with specific residents.

Potential Restorative Nursing Programs

Certification requirements: Range of Motion

A resident who enters the facility without a limited range of motion does not experience a reduction unless the clinical condition demonstrated that it was unavoidable. A resident with a limited range of motion receives appropriate treatment and services to increase and/or prevent further decrease in range of motion.

Range of motion

This is an exercise program of passive and/or active movements to maintain flexibility and useful motion in the joints of the body. *Active range of motion is performed by the resident, with cueing or supervision.

Targeted residents for range of motion include:

- Immobilized

- Bedfast

- Deformities resulting from neurological defects

- Pain, spasms, immobility associated with arthritis

- Late stages of Alzheimer's disease where activity declines

- Limitation in range of impacting on performance ADLs

- Using splints or braces

- Physical restraints

- Side rails for mobility purposes

- Falls, accidents, incontinence

Preventative care may include:

- Active range of motion by resident

- Passive range of motion by staff

- Active assisted range of motion by both

- Application of splints or braces

Splint or brace assistance

A staff member gives verbal and/or physical guidance and direction that teaches the resident how to apply, manipulate, and care for braces or splints. Staff members have a scheduled program of applying and removing the braces/splints, assessing the skin and circulation under the device, and repositioning the limb in a correct alignment.

Resident considerations for splint or brace:

- Residents with spastic paralysis

- Residents with deformity contractures

- Residents with no active range of motion

Goals for splint use:

- Maintain proper alignment of limbs

- Help reduce spasticity

- Provide optimum joint alignment

- Obtain maximum potential range of motion

- Prevent further contractures

Care plan development:

- Include interventions for range of motion

- Provide range of motion prior to application

- Reflect time for pre-care and application

Goals for brace use:

- Prevent foot drop

- Emanate skin pressure on the foot or heels

- Maintain lower leg alignment

Certification requirements: Activities of Daily Living (ADL)

Each resident must receive and the facility must provide the necessary care and services to attain or maintain the highest practical physical, mental, and psychosocial well-being, in accordance with the comprehensive assessment and plan of care.

Based on a comprehensive assessment of the resident, the facility must ensure that the resident's abilities in ADL do not diminish unless circumstances of the individual's clinical condition demonstrate that decline was unavoidable. This includes the ability to bathe, dress, groom, transfer, and ambulate, as well as toilet, eat, and use speech, language, or other functional communication systems.

Restorative programs are targeted at residents who require supervision, limited assist, extensive assist, or total care for any of the ADLs. Restorative programs are indicated for residents who have decision-making ability, and/or if the resident or the staff believes the resident is capable of increased performance. A maintenance program is indicated when the resident has no ability to make decisions and/or has severe limitations caused by medical illness.

ADL training and skill practice

Activities including repetition, physical or verbal cueing, and task segmentation.

Dressing and grooming

Improve or maintain self-performance in dressing, undressing, bathing and washing, and performing personal hygiene tasks.

Targeted residents for mobility programs include:

- Residents with reduced stamina or endurance in physical activities of ambulation, transfer, or positioning

- Residents with stiffening or rigidity of muscles, ligaments, and joints

- Residents with risk factors for negative outcomes:

  - Physical restraints

  - Psychoactive medication

  - Depression

- Residents with a high risk for or history of falls or accidents

Types of programs include:

- Walking/ambulation

- Range of motion

- Strengthening exercises

- Stretching exercises

- Conditioning exercises

- Transfer practice

Bed mobility

Improve or maintain self-performance in moving to and from a lying position, turning side to side, and self-positioning. *Side rails are to be used as intervention for bed mobility; you must evaluate the resident for possible safety risks and take action accordingly.

Transfer

Improve or maintain self-performance in moving between surfaces or planes with/without assistive devices.

Walking

Improve or maintain self-performance in walking with or without assistive devices.

Eating or swallowing

Improve or maintain performance in feeding self food and fluids, or in performing activities to improve/maintain the ability to ingest nutrition and hydration by mouth.

Candidates for a feeding program include:

- Physically disabled residents in need of adaptive equipment

- Residents with mechanically altered diets and a potential for progressive diet behavior modification

- Residents with poor or no use of eating utensils

- Residents exhibiting socially unacceptable or dysfunctional behavior related to eating, meal-time behavior, distractibility, or pacing

Types of programs include:

- Adaptive feeding devices

- Progressive diets

- Utensil training

Amputation/prosthesis care

Improve or maintain self-performance in putting on or taking off or caring for prosthesis.

Communication

Improve or maintain self-performance in using newly acquired functional communication skills or assisting the resident in using residual skills and adaptive equipment.

Certification requirements: Incontinence

A resident who is incontinent of bladder receives appropriate treatment and services to prevent urinary tract infections and to restore as much bladder function as possible. A resident who enters the facility without an indwelling catheter is not catheterized unless the clinical condition demonstrates catheterization was necessary.

Generally, chronic indwelling catheter use should occur only after a restorative program to improve bladder function has been attempted, or after an attempt has been made to manage the incontinence with briefs, padding, scheduled voiding programs, or intermittent catheterization.

Bladder programs

Any scheduled toileting plan: A plan in which the staff, at scheduled times each day, takes the resident to the toilet room, gives the resident a urinal/bedpan, or reminds the resident to go to the bathroom. Includes habit training and prompted voiding programs.

Bladder retraining: Used to manage urinary incontinence due to bladder instability when the resident can be taught to delay or resist the urge to void.

Targeted residents for continence management programs include:

- Residents who are able to be mobilized

- Residents who are able to cooperate

- Residents with functional incontinence

- Residents with stress, urge, or overflow incontinence

Assessment and care planning steps:

- Complete the urinary incontinence RAP

- Complete bladder tracking for 48 to 72 hours

- Develop and implement the care plan

- Track and evaluate results

Bowel training program

Food, fruit, fiber, activity and at least 10 minutes of uninterrupted toilet time are the keys to healthy bowel function!

Targeted residents for bowel training program include:

- Residents who are incontinent of bowel

- Residents triggering dementia/cognitive loss, rehab potential, and insufficient fluids

- Residents with multiple medications to manage bowel function

- Residents with a history of fecal impaction, constipation, poor fluid intakes, poor dietary habits, immobility, or taking iron supplements

Bowel retraining program includes:

- Track bowel habits for 14 days.

- Establish a goal based on the established pattern.

- If no pattern, use laxatives or suppositories to establish a routine. Once established, taper off use. Establishing pattern may take up to three weeks.

- Promote habit by taking the resident to the toilet 30 minutes after suppository is used or after meal or hot liquid is given at a scheduled time. Set aside 10 minutes for this; preferably in an upright position on the toilet.

- Unless contraindicated fluids from 1500 to 2000cc are needed, adding fiber to the diet along with the fluid is most beneficial.

- Encourage and promote exercise and movement on a daily basis, for as long as the resident can tolerate.

Other restorative programs

Residents who present with mental and psychosocial difficulties such as: Impaired communication, social isolation, feelings of powerlessness, undefined anxiety, fear, new admission, grieving, sleep pattern disturbances, negative self-view, aggressive behavior toward self and others, and so forth, may have additional restorative programs developed.

- Teaching self care: Disease management, self administration of medications, ostomy care, cardiac rehab, etc.

- Reality orientation: Substance exposure

- Validation therapy: Meet where they are, not where we are

- Re-motivation: Prompts and encourages involvement

- Adjustment therapy: Acclimates and assists the person in adapting to changes/losses

Clarify Resident Needs and Wants
1. What does the resident want?
2. What is the potential for improving function?
3. Does the resident have the ability to learn?
4. Can he or she call on past memory to solve current problem(s)?
5. What is the general functional status? How disabled? Does status vary?
6. Is mobility severely impaired?
7. Are there behavior problems? Mood problems?
8. Is he or she motivated to work at a restorative program?

Documentation Requirements and Recommendations

The MDS 2.0 section on ADL/Rehabilitation is or can be an initial screen for identifying functional status. The current standard of practice mandated by MDS 2.0 is that residents who are anything less than independent in the performance of ADLs can benefit from a restorative or maintenance ADL program. The type of services and programs that can be of benefit comes out of completing the ADL RAP, which is a required action when triggered by the MDS.

The RUGs or Resource Utilization Groups reimbursement system also recognizes the restorative nursing category in three of the seven primary categories used to classify residents. To group in these classifications it is necessary to provide at least two programs, a minimum of 15 minutes, six days per week. These programs can be maintenance or restorative in nature.

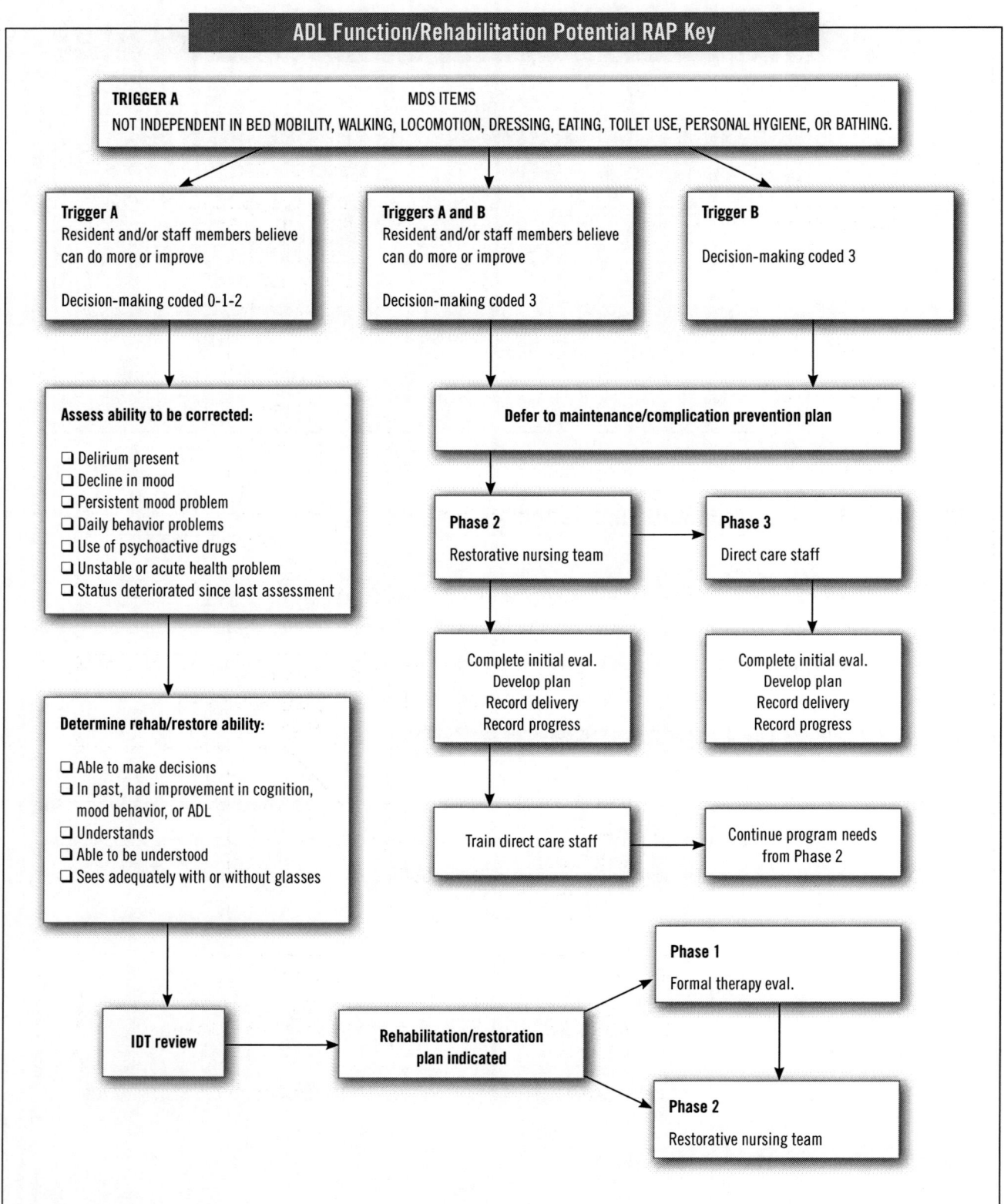

ADL Function/Rehabilitation Potential RAP Key

TRIGGER A — MDS ITEMS
NOT INDEPENDENT IN BED MOBILITY, WALKING, LOCOMOTION, DRESSING, EATING, TOILET USE, PERSONAL HYGIENE, OR BATHING.

Trigger A
Resident and/or staff members believe can do more or improve

Decision-making coded 0-1-2

Triggers A and B
Resident and/or staff members believe can do more or improve

Decision-making coded 3

Trigger B

Decision-making coded 3

Assess ability to be corrected:

❑ Delirium present
❑ Decline in mood
❑ Persistent mood problem
❑ Daily behavior problems
❑ Use of psychoactive drugs
❑ Unstable or acute health problem
❑ Status deteriorated since last assessment

Defer to maintenance/complication prevention plan

Phase 2
Restorative nursing team

Phase 3
Direct care staff

Complete initial eval.
Develop plan
Record delivery
Record progress

Complete initial eval.
Develop plan
Record delivery
Record progress

Determine rehab/restore ability:

❑ Able to make decisions
❑ In past, had improvement in cognition, mood behavior, or ADL
❑ Understands
❑ Able to be understood
❑ Sees adequately with or without glasses

Train direct care staff

Continue program needs from Phase 2

IDT review

Rehabilitation/restoration plan indicated

Phase 1
Formal therapy eval.

Phase 2
Restorative nursing team

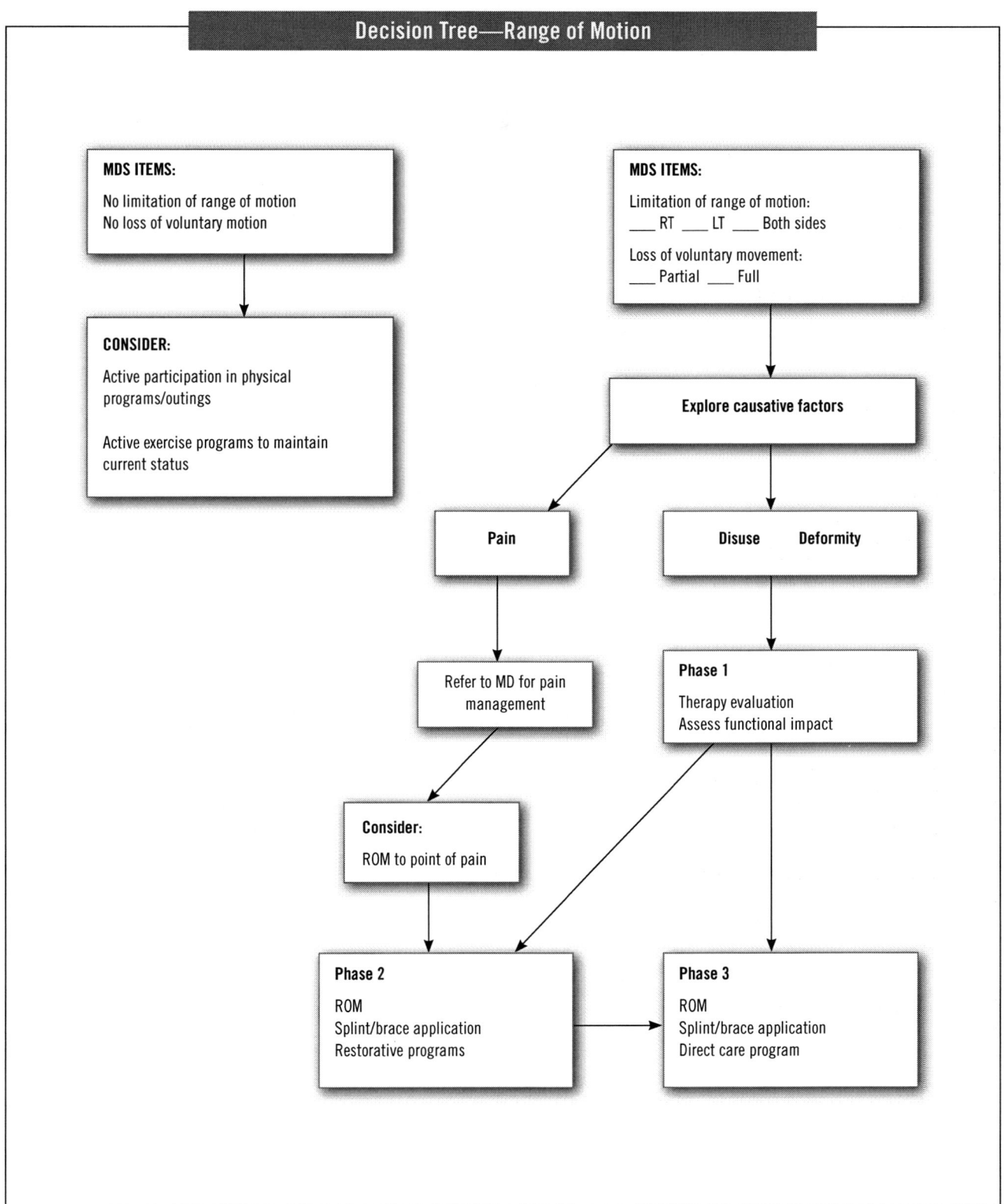

Decision Tree—Range of Motion

MDS ITEMS:

No limitation of range of motion
No loss of voluntary motion

↓

CONSIDER:

Active participation in physical programs/outings

Active exercise programs to maintain current status

MDS ITEMS:

Limitation of range of motion:
____ RT ____ LT ____ Both sides

Loss of voluntary movement:
____ Partial ____ Full

↓

Explore causative factors

Pain

Disuse   Deformity

↓

Refer to MD for pain management

Phase 1

Therapy evaluation
Assess functional impact

↓

Consider:

ROM to point of pain

↓

Phase 2

ROM
Splint/brace application
Restorative programs

Phase 3

ROM
Splint/brace application
Direct care program

Restorative/Maintenance Assessment and Plan: BATHING AND GROOMING

Resident Name: _____   **Date Initiated:** _____

Program Provider: ❑ Restorative Care Staff   ❑ Direct Care Staff

PROBLEM/NEED	GOALS	INTERVENTIONS
Current status:	**Resident will:**	**Skills practice:**
❑ Decision-making = __ 0, 1, 2, __3	❑ Maintain current status	❑ __ 5 __ 10 __ 15 min.
❑ Bathing/grooming = __0, 1, 2, 3, __4	❑ Improve current status	❑ __ days per week
❑ Resident believes can do more		
❑ Staff members believe can do more	**Resident will be able to:**	**Provide:**
❑ Poor attention span	❑ Wet/wring washcloth	❑ Verbal prompts
❑ Distractible	❑ Apply soap	❑ Hands-on support
	❑ Wash face ❑ Wash hands	❑ Task segmentation
Unable to:	❑ Wash upper body	_____
❑ Wet/wring washcloth ❑ Apply soap	❑ Wash lower body ❑ Peri area	_____
❑ Wash face ❑ Wash hands	❑ Dry body parts	_____
❑ Wash upper body	❑ Comb hair ❑ Shave	_____
❑ Wash lower body ❑ Peri area	❑ Apply toothpaste to toothbrush	_____
❑ Dry body parts ❑ Comb hair	❑ Brush teeth	_____
❑ Shave	❑ Remove/insert dentures	_____
❑ Apply toothpaste to brush	❑ Clean dentures	_____
❑ Brush teeth	❑ Clean fingernails	_____
❑ Remove/insert dentures	❑ Apply makeup	_____
❑ Clean dentures	❑ Turn water __ on __ off	_____
❑ Clean fingernails	❑ Physical assist: __ none __ 1 __ 2	_____
❑ Apply makeup		_____
❑ Turn water __ on __ off	**Resident will be:**	_____
❑ Physical assist: __ none __ 1 __ 2	❑ Neat, clean, and well groomed	_____
	❑ _____	_____
Strengths to draw on:	❑ _____	
❑ Follows direction ❑ Understands		❑ See ADL directive
❑ Interested in appearance	**Goal date:** _____	❑ See immediate needs care plan
❑ _____		❑ See core care plan
❑ _____		

Date: _____   ❑ Plan discussed with resident/guardian   ❑ Staff instructed

_____

_____

Signature/Title _____

         The Big Book of Care Plans, Second Edition

Restorative/Maintenance Assessment and Plan: DRESSING

Resident Name: _____ Date Initiated: _____

> Program Provider: ❑ Restorative Care Staff ❑ Direct Care Staff

PROBLEM/NEED	GOALS	INTERVENTIONS
Current status:	**Resident will:**	**Skills practice:**
❑ Decision-making = __ 0, 1, 2, __3	❑ Maintain current status	❑ __ 5 __ 10 __ 15 min.
❑ Dressing = __0, 1, 2, 3, __4	❑ Improve current status	❑ __ days per week
❑ Resident believes can do more		
❑ Staff members believe can do more	**Resident will be able to:**	**Provide:**
❑ Poor attention span	❑ Locate/select clothes	❑ Verbal prompts
	❑ Grasp/put on upper-body clothes	❑ Hands-on support
Unable to:	❑ Grasp/put on lower-body clothes	❑ Task segmentation
❑ Locate/select clothes	❑ Snap snaps	_____
❑ Grasp/put on upper-body clothes	❑ Zip zippers	_____
❑ Grasp/put on lower-body clothes	❑ Button buttons	_____
❑ Snap snaps	❑ Put clothes in correct order	_____
❑ Zip zippers	❑ Remove upper-body clothes	_____
❑ Button buttons	❑ Remove lower-body clothes	_____
❑ Put clothes in correct order	❑ _____	_____
❑ Remove upper-body clothes	❑ _____	_____
❑ Remove lower-body clothes		_____
	Resident will be:	_____
Strengths to draw on:	❑ Appropriately dressed	_____
❑ Follows direction	❑ _____	_____
❑ Interested in appearance	❑ _____	_____
❑ Cooperates		_____
❑ _____	**Goal date:** _____	_____
❑ _____		_____

Needs:		❑ See ADL directive
❑ Rehabilitation/restorative plan		❑ See immediate needs care plan
❑ Maintenance/complication plan		❑ See core care plan

Date: _____ ❑ Plan discussed with resident/guardian ❑ Staff instructed

_____

_____

Signature/Title _____

Restorative/Maintenance Assessment and Plan: EATING/SWALLOWING

Resident Name: _____ Date Initiated: _____

Program Provider: ❑ Restorative Care Staff ❑ Direct Care Staff

PROBLEM/NEED	GOALS	INTERVENTIONS

Current status:

❑ Decision-making = __ 0, __ 1, __ 2, __ 3
❑ Eating = __ 0, __ 1, __ 2, __ 3, __ 4
❑ Resident believes can do more
❑ Staff members believe can do more
❑ Poor attention span
❑ Easily distracted

Unable to:

❑ Swallow ❑ Chew
❑ Use straw
❑ Pick up utensils ❑ Hold utensils
❑ Bring food from plate to mouth
❑ Drink from glass ❑ Drink from covered cup
❑ Open/unwrap __ food __ drinks
❑ Physical assist: __ none __ 1 __ 2

Requires:

❑ Plate guard
❑ Built-up utensils
❑ Specialized drinking cup

Usually eats:

❑ __ 25% __ 50% __ 75% __ 100%

Strengths to draw on:

❑ Stays seated at table
❑ Initiates attempts to feed self
❑ Pays attention to food
❑ _____

Needs:

❑ Rehabilitation/restorative plan
❑ Maintenance/complication plan

Resident will:

❑ Maintain current status
❑ Improve current status

Resident will be able to:

❑ Swallow
❑ Chew
❑ Pick up utensils ❑ Hold utensils
❑ Bring food from plate to mouth
❑ Drink from glass ❑ Drink from covered cup
❑ Open/unwrap __ food __ drinks
❑ Physical assist: __ none __ 1 __ 2
❑ _____
❑ _____

Requires:

❑ Plate guard
❑ Built-up utensils
❑ Specialized drinking cup

Will eat:

❑ __ 25% __ 50% __ 75% __ 100%

Resident will be free of:

❑ Weight loss
❑ Dehydration
❑ Aspiration
❑ _____

Goal date: _____

Skills practice:

❑ __ 5 __ 10 __ 15 min.
❑ __ days per week

Provide:

❑ Verbal prompts
❑ Hands-on support
❑ Task segmentation

_____
_____
_____
_____
_____
_____
_____
_____
_____
_____
_____
_____
_____
_____
_____
_____

❑ See ADL directive
❑ See immediate needs care plan
❑ See core care plan

Date: _____ ❑ Plan discussed with resident/guardian ❑ Staff instructed

_____

_____

Signature/Title _____

Restorative/Maintenance Assessment and Plan: RANGE OF MOTION

Resident Name: _____ Date Initiated: _____

Program Provider: ❑ Restorative Care Staff   ❑ Direct Care Staff

PROBLEM/NEED	GOALS	INTERVENTIONS

Current status:

Functional limitation of:
❑ Neck
❑ Feet: __ RT __ LT __ Bilateral
❑ Arms: __ RT __ LT __ Bilateral
❑ Hands: __ RT __ LT __ Bilateral
❑ Legs: __ RT __ LT __ Bilateral
❑ Other: _____
❑ Voluntary movement
__ No loss __ Partial loss __ Full loss

Due to:
❑ Pain   ❑ Disuse   ❑ Dysfunction

Unable to:
❑ Move self in bed
❑ Propel self in wheelchair
❑ Transfer to/from __ bed __ chair
__ Other: _____
❑ Dress   ❑ Bathe   ❑ Groom
❑ Ambulate

Strengths to draw on:
❑ Cooperates with care
❑ Able to follow direction
❑ _____
❑ _____

Needs:
❑ Rehabilitation/restorative plan
❑ Maintenance/complication plan

Resident will:
❑ Maintain current status
❑ Improve current status

Resident will be able to:
❑ Move self in bed
❑ Propel self in wheelchair
❑ Transfer to/from __ bed __ chair
__ Other: _____
❑ Dress   ❑ Bathe   ❑ Groom
❑ Ambulate
❑ _____
❑ _____
❑ _____

Resident will be free of:
❑ Pain/discomfort
❑ _____
❑ _____
❑ _____

Goal date: _____

Range of motion of affected areas:
❑ __ Active __ Passive __ Active-assistive
❑ __ 5 __ 10 __ 15 min.
❑ __ days per week

Provide:
❑ Verbal prompts
_____
_____
❑ Par trail exercises to/from dining room meals
❑ Sitersize exercise small group by activity staff member
❑ ROM with bathing/grooming
❑ Provide pain medication per MD order
_____
_____
_____
_____
❑ See ADL directive
❑ See immediate needs care plan
❑ See core care plan

Date: _____ ❑ Plan discussed with resident/guardian   ❑ Staff instructed

_____

_____

Signature/Title _____

Restorative/Maintenance Assessment and Plan: RANGE OF MOTION: ARMS AND HANDS

Resident Name: _____ Date Initiated: _____

Program Provider: ❑ Restorative Care Staff ❑ Direct Care Staff

PROBLEM/NEED	GOALS	INTERVENTIONS
Current status:	**Resident will:**	**Range of motion of affected areas:**
❑ Functional limitation of arms, hands	❑ Maintain current status	❑ __ Active __ Passive __ Active-assistive
❑ Voluntary movement of arms, hands	❑ Improve current status	❑ __ 5 __ 10 __ 15 min.
__ No loss __ Partial loss __ Full loss		❑ __ days per week
	Resident will:	
Due to:	❑ Raise arms above head	**Provide:**
❑ Pain ❑ Disuse ❑ Dysfunction	❑ Raise arms straight out from shoulders	❑ Verbal prompts
	❑ Touch top of head	❑ Hand over hand
Unable to:	❑ Touch face	_____
❑ Raise arms above head	❑ Wash upper body	_____
❑ Raise arms straight out from shoulders	❑ Brush teeth	_____
❑ Touch top of head	❑ Comb hair	❑ Dining room meals
❑ Touch face		❑ Sitersize exercise small group by activity
❑ Wash upper body	**Will be free of:**	staff member
❑ Brush teeth	❑ Pain/discomfort	❑ ROM with bathing/grooming
❑ Comb hair	❑ _____	❑ Provide pain medication per MD order
	❑ _____	❑ OT consult as needed
Strengths to draw on:	❑ _____	_____
❑ Cooperates with care		_____
❑ Able to follow direction	**Goal date:** _____	_____
❑ _____		❑ See ADL directive
❑ _____		❑ See immediate needs care plan
		❑ See core care plan

Needs:

❑ Rehabilitation/restorative plan

❑ Maintenance/complication plan

Date: _____ ❑ Plan discussed with resident/guardian ❑ Staff instructed

_____

_____

Signature/Title _____

Restorative/Maintenance Assessment and Plan: RANGE OF MOTION: NECK

Resident Name: _____ Date Initiated: _____

Program Provider: ❑ Restorative Care Staff   ❑ Direct Care Staff

PROBLEM/NEED	GOALS	INTERVENTIONS

Current status:

Resident will:

Range of motion of affected areas:

❑ Functional limitation of neck

❑ Maintain current status

❑ __ Active __ Passive __ Active-assistive

❑ Voluntary movement of neck

❑ Improve current status

❑ __ 5 __ 10 __ 15 min.

__ No loss __ Partial loss __ Full loss

❑ __ days per week

Resident will:

Due to:

❑ Swallow without choking episode

Provide:

❑ Pain   ❑ Disuse   ❑ Dysfunction

❑ _____

❑ Verbal prompts

❑ _____

❑ Hand over hand

Unable to:

❑ _____

❑ Turn head side to side

_____

❑ Tilt head back, chin up

Will be free of:

_____

❑ Tilt head down, chin to chest

❑ Pain/discomfort

❑ Par trail exercises to/from dining room meals

❑ _____

❑ Sitersize exercise small group by activity

Resulting in:

❑ _____

staff member

❑ Difficulty swallowing

❑ ROM with bathing/grooming

❑ Potential for aspiration

Goal date: _____

❑ Provide pain medication per MD order

_____

Strengths to draw on:

_____

❑ Can follow direction

_____

❑ Cooperates with care

_____

❑ _____

❑ _____

❑ See ADL directive

❑ See immediate needs care plan

Needs:

❑ See core care plan

❑ Rehabilitation/restorative plan

❑ Maintenance/complication plan

Date: _____   ❑ Plan discussed with resident/guardian   ❑ Staff instructed

_____

_____

Signature/Title _____

Restorative/Maintenance Assessment and Plan: RANGE OF MOTION: LEGS AND FEET

Resident Name: _____   Date Initiated: _____

Program Provider: ❑ Restorative Care Staff   ❑ Direct Care Staff

PROBLEM/NEED	GOALS	INTERVENTIONS
Current status:	**Resident will:**	**Range of motion of affected areas:**
❑ Functional limitation of arms, hands	❑ Maintain current status	❑ __ Active __ Passive __ Active-assistive
❑ Voluntary movement of legs, feet	❑ Improve current status	❑ __ 5 __ 10 __ 15 min.
__ No loss __ Partial loss __ Full loss		❑ __ days per week
❑ Walks distance of _____ feet	**Will be able to:**	
	❑ Rotate feet in, out	**Provide:**
Due to:	❑ Move feet up and down	❑ Verbal prompts
❑ Pain ❑ Disuse ❑ Dysfunction	❑ Rotate legs in, out	_____
	❑ Move legs up and down	_____
Unable to:	❑ Bear weight	_____
❑ Rotate feet in, out	__ with __ without assistive device	❑ Par trail exercises to/from dining room meals
❑ Move feet up and down	❑ Walk __ to/from bedroom __ to/from dining	❑ Sitersize exercise small group by activity
❑ Rotate legs in, out	room __ outside the facility	staff member
❑ Move legs up and down		❑ ROM with bathing/grooming
❑ Bear weight	**Will be free of:**	❑ Provide pain medication per MD order
__ with __ without assistive device	❑ Pain/discomfort	
❑ Walk __ to/from bedroom __ to/from dining	❑ _____	_____
room __ outside the facility	❑ _____	_____
	❑ _____	_____
Strengths to draw on:		
❑ Can follow direction	**Goal date:** _____	❑ See ADL directive
❑ Cooperates with care		❑ See immediate needs care plan
❑ _____		❑ See core care plan
❑ _____		

Needs:

❑ Rehabilitation/restorative plan

❑ Maintenance/complication plan

Date: _____   ❑ Plan discussed with resident/guardian   ❑ Staff instructed

_____

_____

Signature/Title _____

Restorative/Maintenance Assessment and Plan: RANGE OF MOTION: FEET

Resident Name: _____ Date Initiated: _____

| Program Provider: | ❑ Restorative Care Staff | ❑ Direct Care Staff |

PROBLEM/NEED	GOALS	INTERVENTIONS

Current status:

❑ Functional limitation of feet

❑ Voluntary movement of feet

__ No loss __ Partial loss __ Full loss

Due to:

❑ Pain ❑ Disuse ❑ Dysfunction

Unable to:

❑ Turn feet in, out

❑ Bring feet up toward knees

❑ Place one foot in front of the other

Resulting in:

❑ Unable to bear weight

❑ Unable to walk

❑ _____

Strengths to draw on:

❑ Can follow direction

❑ Cooperates with care

❑ _____

❑ _____

Needs:

❑ Rehabilitation/restorative plan

❑ Maintenance/complication plan

Resident will:

❑ Maintain current status

❑ Improve current status

Will be able to:

❑ Bear weight

❑ Walk

❑ Rotate feet in, out

❑ _____

❑ _____

Will be free of:

❑ Pain/discomfort

❑ _____

❑ _____

Goal date: _____

Range of motion of affected areas:

❑ __ Active __ Passive __ Active-assistive

❑ __ 5 __ 10 __ 15 min.

❑ __ days per week

Provide:

❑ Verbal prompts

_____

_____

_____

❑ Par trail exercises to/from dining room meals

❑ Sitersize exercise small group by activity staff member

❑ ROM with bathing/grooming

❑ Provide pain medication per MD order

❑ PT consult

❑ Apply splint/brace as indicated

_____

_____

_____

❑ See ADL directive

❑ See immediate needs care plan

❑ See core care plan

Date: _____ ❑ Plan discussed with resident/guardian ❑ Staff instructed

_____

_____

Signature/Title _____

Restorative/Maintenance Assessment and Plan: BED MOBILITY

Resident Name: _____ **Date Initiated:** _____

| **Program Provider:** ❑ Restorative Care Staff ❑ Direct Care Staff |

PROBLEM/NEED	GOALS	INTERVENTIONS

Current status:

❑ Decision-making = __ 0, 1, 2, __ 3
❑ Bed mobility = __ 0, 1, 2, 3 __
❑ Resident believes can do more
❑ Staff members believe can do more
❑ Poor attention span
❑ Easily distracted

Unable to:

❑ Move side to side
❑ Sit up in bed from lying down
❑ Position body while in bed
❑ Follow simple commands
❑ Follow complex commands
❑ Needs physical support: __ none __ 1 __ 2

Strengths to draw on:

❑ Upper extremity strength
❑ Recognizes need to change position
❑ _____
❑ _____

Needs:

❑ Rehabilitation/restorative plan
❑ Maintenance/complication plan

Resident will:

❑ Maintain current status
❑ Improve current status

Will be able to:

❑ Move side to side
❑ Sit up in bed from lying down
❑ Position body while in bed
❑ Follow simple commands
❑ Follow complex commands
❑ Needs physical support: __ none __ 1 __ 2

Will be free of:

❑ Pain/discomfort
❑ _____
❑ _____

Goal date: _____

Skills practice:

❑ __ 5 __ 10 __ 15 min.
❑ __ days per week

Provide:

❑ Verbal prompts
❑ Hands-on support
❑ Task segmentation
_____
_____
_____
_____
_____
_____
_____
_____

❑ See ADL directive
❑ See immediate needs care plan
❑ See core care plan

Date: _____ ❑ Plan discussed with resident/guardian ❑ Staff instructed

_____

_____

Signature/Title _____

Restorative/Maintenance Assessment and Plan: TRANSFER

Resident Name: _____ Date Initiated: _____

Program Provider: ❑ Restorative Care Staff ❑ Direct Care Staff

PROBLEM/NEED	GOALS	INTERVENTIONS

Current status:

❑ Decision-making = __ 0, 1, 2, __ 3
❑ Bed mobility = __ 0, 1, 2, 3 __
❑ Resident believes can do more
❑ Staff members believe can do more
❑ Poor attention span
❑ Distractible

Unable to:
❑ Turn side to side
❑ Lift legs off bed
❑ Move to/from bed
❑ Move from sitting to standing
❑ Move to/from WC/chair

Balance is:
❑ Steady   ❑ Unsteady
❑ Needs physical support: __ none __ 1 __ 2

Mode of transfer is:
❑ Bedrails
❑ Transfer aide _____
❑ Bedfast
❑ Lifted manually with assist: __ 1 __ 2
❑ Lifted mechanically

Strengths to draw on:
❑ Follows direction
❑ Cooperates with care
❑ _____

Needs:
❑ Rehabilitation/restorative plan
❑ Maintenance/complication plan

Resident will:
❑ Maintain current status
❑ Improve current status

Will be able to:
❑ Turn side to side
❑ Lift legs off bed
❑ Move to/from bed
❑ Move from sitting to standing
❑ Move to/from WC/chair
❑ Physical assist of: __ 1 __ 2

Balance will be:
❑ Steady   ❑ Unsteady
❑ Physical assist of: __ 1 __ 2

Mode of transfer will be:
❑ Bedrails
❑ Transfer aide _____
❑ Lifted manually with assist: __ 1 __ 2
❑ Lifted mechanically

Will be free of:
❑ Pressure ulcers
❑ Falls
❑ _____

Goal date: _____

Skills practice:

❑ __ 5 __ 10 __ 15 min.
❑ __ days per week

Provide:
❑ Verbal prompts
❑ Hands-on support
❑ Use gait belt
❑ Shoes on securely
❑ Task segmentation

_____
_____
_____
_____
_____
_____
_____
_____
_____
_____
_____
_____

❑ See ADL directive
❑ See immediate needs care plan
❑ See core care plan

Date: _____ ❑ Plan discussed with resident/guardian ❑ Staff instructed

_____
_____

Signature/Title _____

Restorative/Maintenance Assessment and Plan: WALKING

Resident Name: _____ Date Initiated: _____

Program Provider: ❑ Restorative Care Staff   ❑ Direct Care Staff

PROBLEM/NEED	GOALS	INTERVENTIONS

Current status:

❑ Decision-making = __ 0, __ 1, __ 2, __ 3
❑ Locomotion = __ 0, __ 1, __ 2, __ 3
❑ Resident believes can do more
❑ Staff members believe can do more
❑ Poor attention span

Unable to:
❑ Walk in room
❑ Walk in corridor
❑ Walk in bathroom
❑ Walk to dining room
❑ Take few steps
❑ Negotiate steps

Balance is:
❑ Steady   ❑ Unsteady
❑ Needs physical support: __ none __ 1 __ 2

Requires assistive device:
❑ Hand rail   ❑ Gait belt
❑ Walker __ Wheels __ No wheels
❑ Cane __ Straight __ Multiple prong
❑ Parallel bars

Strengths to draw on:
❑ Cooperates with care
❑ Attempts to ambulate on own
❑ Can follow direction
❑ _____

Needs:
❑ Rehabilitation/restorative plan
❑ Maintenance/complication plan

Resident will:

❑ Maintain current status
❑ Improve current status

Resident will be able to:
❑ Walk in room with assist of:
__ none __ 1 __ 2
❑ Walk in corridor with assist of:
__ none __ 1 __ 2
❑ Number of feet _____
❑ For _____ minutes
❑ _____

Balance will be:
❑ Steady
❑ With physical support: __ none __ 1 __ 2

Will be free of:
❑ Falls
❑ _____
❑ _____

Goal date: _____

Skills practice:

❑ __ 5 __ 10 __ 15 min.
❑ __ days per week

Provide:
❑ Verbal prompts
❑ Hands-on support
❑ Use of gait belt
❑ Use of cane
❑ Use of walker
❑ Task segmentation
❑ Sitersize exercise small group by activity staff member
❑ Par trail exercises to/from dining room meals

_____
_____
_____
_____
_____
_____
_____
_____
_____
_____
_____

❑ See ADL directive
❑ See immediate needs care plan
❑ See core care plan

Date: _____   ❑ Plan discussed with resident/guardian   ❑ Staff instructed

_____

_____

Signature/Title _____

Restorative/Maintenance Assessment and Plan: WHEELCHAIR MOBILITY

Resident Name: _____   **Date Initiated:** _____

Program Provider: ❏ Restorative Care Staff   ❏ Direct Care Staff

PROBLEM/NEED	GOALS	INTERVENTIONS

Current status:

❏ Decision-making = __ 0, 1, 2, __ 3
❏ Locomotion = __ 0, 1, 2, 3 __ 4
❏ Resident believes can do more
❏ Staff members believe can do more
❏ Poor attention span

Unable to:
❏ Propel wheelchair: __ In room __ In corridor
__ To bathroom __ Throughout the facility
❏ Transfer self to wheelchair
❏ Self-propel short distance, _____ feet
❏ Self-propel long distance, _____ feet

Sitting balance is:
❏ Steady   ❏ Unsteady
❏ Needs physical support: __ none __ 1 __ 2

Strengths to draw on:
❏ Able to follow direction
❏ Desires to be out of the room daily
❏ Understands
❏ _____

Needs:
❏ Rehabilitation/restorative plan
❏ Maintenance/complication plan

Resident will:

❏ Maintain current status
❏ Improve current status

Will be able to:
❏ Transfer self and propel chair with assist of:
__ none __ 1 __ 2
❏ Propel in corridor with assist of:
__ none __ 1 __ 2
❏ Propel to bathroom __ and back __ with
assist of: __ none __ 1 __ 2
❏ Propel to dining room __ and back __ with
assist of: __ none __ 1 __ 2
❏ Distance: maximum feet _____ in _____ min.

Sitting balance will be:
❏ Steady
❏ _____

Will be free of:
❏ Falls
❏ _____
❏ _____

Goal date: _____

Skills practice:

❏ __ 5 __ 10 __ 15 min.
❏ __ days per week

Provide:
❏ Verbal prompts
❏ Hands-on support
❏ Task segmentation
❏ Par trail exercises to/from dining room meals
❏ Sitersize exercise small group by activity
staff member
_____
_____
_____
_____
_____
_____
_____
_____
_____
_____
_____
_____

❏ See ADL directive
❏ See immediate needs care plan
❏ See core care plan

Date: _____   ❏ Plan discussed with resident/guardian   ❏ Staff instructed

_____

_____

Signature/Title _____

Restorative/Maintenance Assessment and Plan: SPLINT/BRACE

Resident Name: _____ **Date Initiated:** _____

Program Provider: ❑ Restorative Care Staff ❑ Direct Care Staff

PROBLEM/NEED	GOALS	INTERVENTIONS
Current status:	**Resident will:**	**Skills practice:**
❑ Muscle tone: __ Spastic __ Flaccid	❑ Maintain current status	❑ __ 5 __ 10 __ 15 min.
❑ Feet: __ RT __ LT __ Bilateral	❑ Improve current status	❑ __ days per week
❑ Arms: __ RT __ LT __ Bilateral		
❑ Hands: __ RT __ LT __ Bilateral	**Resident will be able to:**	**Provide:**
❑ Legs: __ RT __ LT __ Bilateral	❑ Move self in bed	❑ Verbal prompts
	❑ Propel self in wheelchair	❑ Hand over hand
Due to:	❑ Transfer to/from __ bed __ chair	❑ ROM to affected extremity prior to application
❑ Disuse	__ other _____	❑ Follow on/off schedule as indicated
❑ Dysfunction	❑ Dress ❑ Bathe ❑ Groom	__ ADL directive __ posted schedule
	❑ Ambulate	_____
Unable to:	❑ _____	_____
❑ Move self in bed	❑ _____	_____
❑ Propel self in wheelchair	❑ _____	_____
❑ Transfer to/from __ bed __ chair		_____
__ other _____	**Will be free of:**	_____
❑ Dress ❑ Bathe ❑ Groom	❑ Pain/discomfort	_____
❑ Ambulate	❑ Contractures	_____
	❑ _____	_____
Strengths to draw on:		_____
❑ Cooperates with care	**Goal date:** _____	_____
❑ Follows direction		_____
❑ _____		_____
❑ _____		_____
		_____
Needs:		_____
❑ Rehabilitation/restorative plan		❑ See ADL directive
❑ Maintenance/complication plan		❑ See immediate needs care plan
		❑ See core care plan

Date: _____ ❑ Plan discussed with resident/guardian ❑ Staff instructed

_____

_____

Signature/Title _____

Rehabilitation Grooming Evaluation

Resident: _____ **Date:** _____

I = Independent **S** = Supervision **LA** = Limited Assist **EA** = Extensive Assist **TD** = Total Dependence

Function	I	S	LA	EA	TD	Comments
Wash face						
Dry face						
Wash hands						
Dry hands						
Shave						
Comb hair						
Apply toothpaste to toothbrush						
Brush teeth						
Remove/insert dentures						
Clean dentures						
Clean mouth with swab						
Clean fingernails						
Apply makeup						

Summary Statement of Problem/Need:

_____

_____

_____

_____

_____

_____

_____

_____

Refer to: OT _____   Nursing Restorative _____   Direct Care Staff _____

Signature/Title: _____

Feeding Evaluation

Resident: _____ Date: _____

I = Independent   S = Supervision   LA = Limited Assist   EA = Extensive Assist   TD = Total Dependence

Function	I	S	LA	EA	TD	Comments
Current feeding status						
Ability to bring food from plate to mouth						

Other considerations	Yes	No	Comments
Eats all meals without tiring			
Eats 50% of all meals			
Eats 25% or less of all meals			
Hand tremors present			
Poor coordination			
Easily distracted/poor attention span			
Unable to hold utensils			
Positioning problems			
Adaptive feeding devices required			
Gags/difficulty swallowing			
Spits out food			

Summary Statement of Problem/Need:

_____

_____

_____

_____

_____

_____

_____

Refer to: OT _____   Nursing Restorative _____   Direct Care Staff _____

Signature/Title: _____

Rehabilitation Transfer/Ambulation Evaluation

Resident: _____ Date: _____

I = Independent   S = Supervision   LA = Limited Assist   EA = Extensive Assist   TD = Total Dependence

Function	I	S	LA	EA	TD	Comments
Turn side to side in bed						
Move from lying to sitting						
Move from sitting to standing						
Bend knees						
Move from bed to chair						
Move from dangle position						
Putting shoes/socks on and off						
Use of cane/walker						
Walk in room						
Walk in facility						
Mobilize wheelchair						
Balance self						

Summary Statement of Problem/Need:

_____

_____

_____

_____

_____

_____

_____

Refer to: OT _____   Nursing Restorative _____   Direct Care Staff _____

Signature/Title: _____

Urinary Incontinence RAP Guidelines

Purpose: Identify reversible causes, minimize occurrence, maintain dignity

Resident name: _____ Date: _____ Evaluator/Title: _____

❏ High Risk Incontinence (Dependent in mobility and/or severe cognitive impairment) ❏ Low Risk for Incontinence is all others incontinent

Directions: After responding to ALL items, review the information and determine the KEY ISSUES AND STRENGTHS. This becomes the basis for your analysis of whether to proceed to care planning.

CONSIDERATIONS	YES	NO	CLARIFICATIONS
1. Conditions Urinary tract infection ruled out ❏ U/A done ❏ C&S done ❏ Pain urination/bladder			
Bowel impaction ruled out ❏ Rectal exam done and results negative			
Delirium present Acute confusional state			
Exhibits signs of depression Symptoms noted on MDS			
2. Concurrent Medical Problems ❏ Diabetes ❏ High blood glucose			
❏ CHF ❏ CVA ❏ Parkinson's			
❏ Edema			
❏ Recurrent UTIs ❏ Fecal impactions			
Dementia ❏ No awareness of urges ❏ Some awareness ❏ Can respond to urges ❏ Can cooperate in toileting			
Cancer ❏ Bladder ❏ Prostate ❏ Brain ❏ Spine			
3. Environment/Functional Status Requires help to transfer			
Distances or problems getting to toilet			
Timely access to toilet			
Able to find the toilet facilities			
Can cooperate with toileting			
Able to manage clothing			
Able to wipe self			
Aware of urge to void (at least some of the time)			
Restraints used			
Side rails used			
4. Medications ❏ Diuretics ❏ Urine output > liter/day ❏ Urine output < liter/day			
❏ Disopyramide ❏ Antispasmodics			
❏ Sympathomimetics ❏ Beta blockers			
❏ Ca channel blockers ❏ Parkinson's med.			
❏ Antipsychotics ❏ Antianxiety/hypnotics			
❏ Antidepressants ❏ Narcotics			
5. Abnormal Labs ❏ High blood calcium ❏ Low B$_{12}$			
❏ High bun ❏ High creatine			
6. Bladder Tracking Results ❏ Pattern to voiding ❏ No pattern established			
7. Type of Incontinence ❏ Stress Incont. ❏ Urge Incont. ❏ Overflow ❏ Functional ❏ Neurogenic bladder			

The Big Book of Care Plans, Second Edition

Bladder Tracking for MDS PLUS

Resident: _____ **Date:** _____ **to** _____

Code directions: In each two-hour time period, mark the code that best describes the status. Use this as a tracking record to determine bowel and bladder habits.

I = Incontinent when checked   **X** = Out of facility at the time or sleeping

CODE:
1 = Taken/prompted and voided; resident unaware of need
2 = Taken/prompted and did not void; resident unaware of need
3 = Taken, dry and then incontinent in that time period
4 = Self-control, voided
5 = Self-control with assistance
6 = Self-control dry, did not need to void in that time period

* Record I = 0 q2h x 3 days.
* Review relationship of I = 0 to any incontinence patterns

Compare relationship of incontinence to times of intake and meals to see whether the pattern emerges. Residents usually need to toilet after meals, first thing in the morning, and HS.

Day	1	I+0	2	I+0	3	I+0	
7 a.m. to 9 a.m.							
9 a.m. to 11 a.m.							
11 a.m. to 1 p.m.							
1 p.m. to 3 p.m.							
3 p.m. to 5 p.m.							
5 p.m. to 7 p.m.							
7 p.m. to 9 p.m.							
9 p.m. to 11 p.m.							
11 p.m. to 1 a.m.							
1 a.m. to 3 a.m.							
3 a.m. to 5 a.m.							
5 a.m. to 7 a.m.							

Bowel habits: I = Incontinent   S = Self-control   Code and note time of occurrence

Restorative Care Plan: URINARY INCONTINENCE

Name: _____   Date Initiated: _____

PROBLEM/NEED	GOALS	INTERVENTIONS

PROBLEM/NEED

Types of incontinence

❏ Functional
   ❏ Physical   ❏ Mental   ❏ Both

❏ Urge incontinence (abrupt loss of urine)

❏ Overflow incontinence (constant dribble)

❏ Stress incontinence (spurts of urine)

❏ Obstruction or stricture

❏ Unable to determine

❏ Other: _____

Aware of urge to void
❏ Yes   ❏ No   ❏ Occasionally

Can cooperate with toileting
❏ Yes   ❏ No   ❏ Occasionally

Mobility status:
❏ Indep.   ❏ Supervised   ❏ Assist
❏ Dependent

Able to manage clothing
❏ Yes   ❏ No

Able to wipe self
❏ Yes   ❏ No

GOALS

❏ Independent continence (continent on own)

❏ Dependent continence
   (continent thru efforts of others)

❏ Social continence (clean, dry, odor-free)

❏ Incontinent episodes < 1x/week
   (usually will be continent)

❏ 2x/week or > but not daily
   (only occasionally incontinent)

INTERVENTIONS

❏ **Habit Training:** No pattern established.
Toilet every _____
                  Day   Eves   Nites
Clean and change if needed.

❏ **Scheduled:** Based on voiding pattern
Toilet every _____
                  Day   Eves   Nites
Clean and change if needed.

❏ **Prompted:** Occ/always aware of need
Toilet every _____
                  Day   Eves   Nites
Clean and change if needed.

❏ **Check and Change** / P&P
Toilet every _____
                  Day   Eves   Nites

❏ Bladder retraining protocol

❏ SEE ALSO RESTORATIVE
   NURSING PROGRAM FOR:

_____

_____

Goal date: _____

Date: _____   ❏ Plan discussed with resident/guardian   ❏ Staff instructed

_____

_____

Signature/Title _____

The Big Book of Care Plans, Second Edition

Restorative Care Plan, Delivery Record, and Progress Notes

❑ Restorative Nursing Plan   **PROGRAM PLAN:** _____
❑ Direct Care Staff Plan

This form is completed by restorative nurse or care coordinator.

Name: _____ **Date of initiation:** _____

Problem/Need statement/Date: _____
_____
_____

Goal: _____
_____

Intervention: _____
_____
_____

Signature/Title/Date: _____

Month: _____ **Year:** _____   ❑ 5 minutes   ❑ 10 minutes   ❑ 15 minutes   ❑ _____ minutes

TREATMENT COMPONENT	1	2	3	4	5	6	7	8	9	10	11	12	13	14	15	16	17	18	19	20	21	22	23	24	25	26	27	28	29	30	31
❑ 7–3																															
❑ 3–11																															
❑ 11–7																															

PROVIDER NAME	TITLE	INITIAL	PROVIDER NAME	TITLE	INITIAL
1.					
2.					
3.			**CODE: R** = PT refused **W** = Treatment withheld – Reason noted		
INITIAL WHEN TREATMENT GIVEN			**I** = Patient Ill **O** = Other appointment		

Progress note: _____
_____
_____
_____

Signature/Title/Date: _____

Restorative Care Plan, Delivery Record, and Progress Notes (cont.)

Program title: _____

Directions: The care plan section is to be completed by a licensed nurse. The delivery records are to be completed following the delivery of service. Progress notes are completed per policy.

Resident name: _____ **Date of initiation:** _____

Functional Problem/Need	Goal(s)	Interventions ❑ Restorative Nursing ❑ Direct Care
	❑ Improve functional status _____ _____ ❑ Maintain functional status _____ _____ ❑ Minimize decline ❑ Prevent complications of: _____	Program to be delivered minimum of 15 minutes/day six days/week.
	Goal Date: _____	**Developed By:** _____

Month: _____ **Year:** _____

TREATMENT COMPONENT	1	2	3	4	5	6	7	8	9	10	11	12	13	14	15	16	17	18	19	20	21	22	23	24	25	26	27	28	29	30	31
❑ 7–3																															
❑ 3–11																															
❑ 11–7																															

PROVIDER NAME	TITLE	INITIAL	PROVIDER NAME	TITLE	INITIAL
1.					
2.					
3.			**CODE: R** = PT refused	**W** = Treatment withheld – Reason noted	
INITIAL WHEN TREATMENT GIVEN			**I** = Patient Ill	**O** = Other appointment	

Progress note: _____
_____
_____
_____

Signature/Title/Date: _____

Restorative Care Plan, Delivery Record, and Progress Notes (cont.)

Restorative Delivery Record for: _____

❑ Restorative Nursing Plan   ❑ Direct Care Staff Plan

Resident name: _____   **Date initiated:** _____

PROVIDER NAME	TITLE	INITIAL	PROVIDER NAME	TITLE	INITIAL
1.					
2.					
3.			**CODE: R** = PT refused **W** = Treatment withheld – Reason noted		
INITIAL WHEN TREATMENT GIVEN			**I** = Patient Ill **O** = Other appointment		

Month: _____ **Year:** _____ ❑ 5 minutes   ❑ 10 minutes   ❑ 15 minutes   ❑ _____ minutes

TREATMENT COMPONENT	1	2	3	4	5	6	7	8	9	10	11	12	13	14	15	16	17	18	19	20	21	22	23	24	25	26	27	28	29	30	31

Progress note: _____
_____
_____

Signature/Title/Date: _____

Month: _____ **Year:** _____ ❑ 5 minutes   ❑ 10 minutes   ❑ 15 minutes   ❑ _____ minutes

TREATMENT COMPONENT	1	2	3	4	5	6	7	8	9	10	11	12	13	14	15	16	17	18	19	20	21	22	23	24	25	26	27	28	29	30	31

Progress note: _____
_____
_____

Signature/Title/Date: _____

Restorative Care Plan, Delivery Record, and Progress Notes (cont.)

❏ Restorative Nursing Plan ❏ Direct Care Staff Plan **Restorative Delivery Record for:** _____

Resident name: _____ **Date initiated:** _____

PROVIDER NAME	TITLE	INITIAL	PROVIDER NAME	TITLE	INITIAL
1.					
2.					
3.			**CODE: R** = PT refused **W** = Treatment withheld – Reason noted		
INITIAL WHEN TREATMENT GIVEN			**I** = Patient Ill **O** = Other appointment		

Month: _____ **Year:** _____ ❏ 5 minutes ❏ 10 minutes ❏ 15 minutes ❏ _____ minutes

TREATMENT COMPONENT	1	2	3	4	5	6	7	8	9	10	11	12	13	14	15	16	17	18	19	20	21	22	23	24	25	26	27	28	29	30	31
❏ 7–3																															
❏ 3–11																															
❏ 11–7																															
TX UNIT = #																															

Month: _____ **Year:** _____ 1RX UNIT = ❏ 5 minutes ❏ 10 minutes ❏ 15 minutes ❏ _____ minutes

TREATMENT COMPONENT	1	2	3	4	5	6	7	8	9	10	11	12	13	14	15	16	17	18	19	20	21	22	23	24	25	26	27	28	29	30	31
❏ 7–3																															
❏ 3–11																															
❏ 11–7																															
TX UNIT = #																															

Month: _____ **Year:** _____ 1RX UNIT = ❏ 5 minutes ❏ 10 minutes ❏ 15 minutes ❏ _____ minutes

TREATMENT COMPONENT	1	2	3	4	5	6	7	8	9	10	11	12	13	14	15	16	17	18	19	20	21	22	23	24	25	26	27	28	29	30	31
❏ 7–3																															
❏ 3–11																															
❏ 11–7																															
❏ 7–3																															
TX UNIT = #																															

Month: _____ **Year:** _____ 1RX UNIT = ❏ 5 minutes ❏ 10 minutes ❏ 15 minutes ❏ _____ minutes

Progress Notes

Additional Restorative Progress Notes for: _____

❑ Restorative Nursing Plan   ❑ Direct Care Staff Plan

Resident name: _____

Progress note: _____
_____
_____
_____

Signature/Title/Date: _____

Progress note: _____
_____
_____
_____

Signature/Title/Date: _____

Progress note: _____
_____
_____
_____

Signature/Title/Date: _____

Progress note: _____
_____
_____
_____

Signature/Title/Date: _____

Progress note: _____
_____
_____
_____

Signature/Title/Date: _____

Restorative Delivery Record

Program: _____

Resident name: _____ **Date initiated:** _____

Directions: Using the key below complete delivery record following program delivery. If resident refuses program or complains of pain or discomfort notify the restorative nurse or RN responsible for care. Use the progress note on the reverse side for comments, particularly if problems are noted or anything unusual has occurred.

Key:

Participation	**C** = Cooperative	**U** = Uncooperative	**R** = Refused		
How tolerated	**W** = Well	**P** = Poor	**O** = Other *(requires a note)*		
Level of assistance provided	**I** = Independent	**S** = Supervised/standby	**LA** = Limited assistance	**EA** = Extensive assistance	**D** = Dependent

SERVICE TO BE PROVIDED: See plan attached or _____

		2	3	4	5	6	7	8	9	10	11	12	13	14	15	16	17	18	19	20	21	22	23	24	25	26	27	28	29	30	31
Minutes of service delivered																																
Participation																																
Tolerance																																
Level of assistance																																
Provider initials																																

Signature/Title	Initials	Signature/Title	Initials

MDS Clinical Pathways

MDS Clinical Pathways: Introduction

We all know the importance of an accurate, timely minimum data set (MDS) for certification, reimbursement, and, more importantly, the delivery of quality care. The pathways in this manual emphasize a truly holistic, interdisciplinary approach to care planning. The pathways eliminate the piecemeal approach to MDS completion, which emphasizes a paper environment. The role of the RN assessment coordinator is shifted from checking MDS sections for completion (which was multidisciplinary, redundant, and wasted time) to assimilating data from multiple sources, thus providing holistic (interdisciplinary, effective, accurate) responses on the MDS. The pathways are designed to focus clinical attention on the resident while ensuring collected information supports MDS coding.

The pathways provide a framework for initiating and completing the MDS, resident assessment protocol (RAP), and care planning processes. Separate pathways are developed to address admission, significant status change, and quarterly and annual reviews. Additional pathways are presented to deal with Medicare prospective payment system demands.

These pathways are guidelines. While they can be implemented as written, a facility may choose to modify and/or rearrange tasks, responsibilities, and time frames to address their individual circumstances or preferences more effectively.

Use of these pathways is at the sole desecration of the purchaser. Regulatory requirements are always subject to change. User assumes full responsibility for use and implementation.

Non-Medicare Admission Assessment Procedure

The pathway has been developed using day 10 as the assessment reference date. If a different reference date is chosen, adjust the pathway accordingly.

A comprehensive assessment must always be completed within 14 days of admission to the facility. A comprehensive assessment consists of the MDS, triggered RAPs, and professional assessments. To ensure consistent and accurate information the Assessment Reference Date for the MDS is established as day 10 for all new non-Medicare admissions.

Re-admissions do not require a new MDS unless there has been a significant status change, the absence from the facility has been greater than _____ days, or a resident who was discharged without the expectation for return is re-admitted.

1. MDS Assessment Reference Date (ARD) will be day 10 of admission (counting day of admission as day one). All professional assessments must be completed and on the chart by the MDS Assessment Reference Date. This enables the RN responsible for care to consider all data prior to responding to the MDS items. Data collection and any tracking tools are to be given to the Registered Nurse Assessment Coordinator (RNAC) the day following the Assessment Reference Date, as the reference date is the last day of data collection. Professional assessments are initiated and completed in timelines indicated on the admission pathway. If assessments cannot be completed in these time frames, a progress note will be written to explain the reason for the delay. Arrangements will be made with the RN responsible for care to ensure the MDS is completed accurately, in a timely manner. The RN responsible for care will distribute data collection tools to nurses and aides preceding the MDS ARD, as noted on the admission pathway. At a minimum, this consists of mood/behavior, ADL data collection, and fall- and skin-risk RAP assessments.

2. RNAC will review data and the professional assessments, completing MDS items in a holistic manner. If conflicts or discrepancies exist, clarification must be sought prior to completing the information. Complete the MDS at least 48 hours prior to the scheduled end date. This will allow time to review MDS coding and insure all triggered RAPs have been addressed.

3. The MDS end date is ALWAYS day 14, including day one of admission. The RAP summary sheet and all triggered RAPs are now completed.

4. All disciplines are to review the completed MDS PRIOR to care conference and BEFORE the MDS is locked. Develop a worksheet on contents, including pertinent information from the professional assessment. Create a problem/needs list for care conference. Professional disciplines will care plan prior to, or at, care conferences, depending on the nature of the identified problems and needs. Disciplines are to come to conference prepared to participate, problem solve, and finalize the care plan. The care conference will be scheduled between day 14 and day 21 following MDS completion.

5. At conferences, write a team note. The intention of this note is to "tie up" the loose ends and bring the pieces together, summarizing the plan and actions to be taken. All team members sign the note, indicating consensus. It is NOT necessary to write the contents of the care plan or RAPs here. Referencing the care plan and RAPs is sufficient.

Assessment Pathway: Admission Assessment and Care Plan

The MDS, triggered RAPs, professional assessments, and ADL and mood/behavior tracking tools make up the admission assessment. The resident assessment must be completed within 14 days of admission. The day of admission is considered day one. The care plan is also initiated on day one to address immediate needs, predominantly of a medical/nursing nature or significant psychosocial concern. It is completed no later than seven days after the end date of the MDS.

RNAC = Resident Nurse Assessment Coordinator   CN = Any licensed nurse

Day 1		
TASK	**RESPONSIBILITY**	**ACTIONS**
Nursing assessment including RAP guidelines for vision, communication, and dental	Admitting nurse	Review transfer records, orders, examine resident. Complete nursing assessment.
Pressure ulcer RAP risk assessment Fall RAP risk assessment	Charge nurse	RNAC assigns to CN, CN completes and initiates plan of care (POC) insert if risk is present.
Physical restraint RAP (before accepting order)	Charge nurse/RNAC	Complete the RAP before taking or requesting orders for restraint use.
Psychoactive drug RAP (can be moved to 2 or 3 on the path)	Charge nurse/RNAC	If ordered, assigned CN collects data, RNAC analyzes and validates decisions on back of form.
Immediate needs care plan (INPOC) and nurse's notes	Charge nurse	Plans are to be initiated for pertinent diagnosis, treatments, behaviors, and mood concerns. Nurse's note frequency is to be reflected on the companion note accompanying the INPOC.
Admission nursing notes	Charge nurse all shifts x 72 hrs **Note:** Frequency and duration are dependent on facility. Adjust path accordingly.	Address general status and adjustment to the facility, actions initiated/completed, notifications, appetite, sleep patterns, etc.

	Day 2	

TASK	RESPONSIBILITY	ACTIONS
Review orders, assessments, resident status, and needs	RNAC	Review chart, orders, diagnosis, and meds. Visit with resident, assessing further if indicated. Validate accuracy of nursing assessment. Ensure dental, vision, and communication RAP data are complete. **Note:** Complete the analysis/decision-making as needed, signing the appropriate section. Make any needed referrals to other disciplines. If conditions warrant, contact other disciplines to initiate assessments sooner than pathway indicates.
If signs and symptoms of delirium are present: Complete delirium RAP	RNAC	By end of Day 4: Initiate standalone delirium RAP, analyze information, and proceed accordingly.
Initiate dietary assessment and RAP review for nutrition, hydration, and tube feeding **Note:** RNAC will be responding to time-sensitive ARD information on the MDS using tracking tools and flow records. If there is a discrepancy of significance due to time-related data, a team note or an episodic progress note can be written to clarify.	Dietitian or dietary tech **Note:** This will depend on policy and specific needs of resident. The dietitian will always review tech findings.	By Day 5: Complete assessment and RAP review for nutrition, hydration, tube feedings. Validate decisions for care planning. Review immediate needs POC, add or contribute as needed. Initiate CORE plan for nutrition, hydration, and tube feeding, if indicated, in preparation for conference.

Day 3		
TASK	**RESPONSIBILITY**	**ACTIONS**
Begin ADL and mood/behavior tracking records **Note:** The day this is initiated is based on ARD. This path assumes day 10 as ARD. Move on path to accommodate ARD time period.	Nurse aide/charge nurse	RNAC provides forms, instructs CN, who will interview NA at end of each shift and complete documents day 3–9. CN collects data end of each shift x 7 days. RNAC collects data on Day 10.
Initiate social history, assessment, and RAP review for cognition, mood, behavior, and well being	Social service	By Day 7: Review record, interview resident, family, staff. If needed, expand assessment via use of mini-status exam, geri-depression scale, etc. Complete assessment and make care planning decisions. Review immediate needs POC; add or contribute as needed. Initiate core plan for cognition, mood, behavior, and well being, if indicated, in preparation for conference.
"Getting to know you conference" (Day 3 to 5)	Resident, family, RNAC, social service	Discuss resident, family concerns, fears. Obtain needed data.

Day 4		
TASK	**RESPONSIBILITY**	**ACTIONS**
Admission nursing notes completed	Charge nurse	Nurse's notes from this point on will be done based on immediate needs care plans and on an episodic basis as the need arises.

 The Big Book of Care Plans, Second Edition

Day 5

TASK	RESPONSIBILITY	ACTIONS
Initiate activity assessment and activity RAP review	Activity staff	By Day 8: Review record, interview resident, family, staff. Complete assessment and validate care planning decisions. Determine if activity interventions are needed on immediate needs POC, adding if pertinent. Ensure resident has needs/preferences acted on if possible. Initiate core plan for activities if indicated. This may wait until professional conference unless vital.
Dietary assessment completed. "Getting to know you" conference completed.	Dietary	Care planning needs considered and formulated.
If incontinent Initiate incontinence RAP Initiate B&B, I&O tracker	RNAC or designated restorative nurse Charge nurse/nurse aide	Days 5–7: RNAC begins data collection for RAP. RNAC gives CN trackers. CN instructs aide to complete during the shift. CN/NA reviews tracker for completion at end of shift.

Day 7

TASK	RESPONSIBILITY	ACTIONS
Social service assessment and RAPs completed	Social services	Care planning needs considered and formulated.

Day 8

TASK	RESPONSIBILITY	ACTIONS
B&B/I&O tracking completed	CN/NA	
Complete incontinence RAP analysis	RNAC or designated restorative nurse	Analyze RAP data. Confer with pharmacy, physician, rehab, and restorative care as needed.
Initiate management program		Implement continence management program.
		Instruct CN to complete daily incontinence nurse's notes x 7 days, then weekly x 4.
Activity RAP and assessment completed	Activities	Care planning needs considered and formulated.

Day 10

TASK	RESPONSIBILITY	ACTIONS
ADL, mood and behavior; B&B, I&O tracking completed	CN	RNAC collects reviews and clarifies.
MDS ARD	Data entry	Open MDS.
	RNAC	Initiate MDS document, complete responses by Day 12.
		- Review all professional assessments, tracking records, medication, and treatment records.
		- Examine resident.
		- Make holistic responses on MDS document.
ADL directives care plan formalized	RNAC	RNAC assists CN to complete, review with nursing assistants on all shifts for accuracy.
	CN/NA	Ensure ADL directives reflect restorative service needs from ADL RAP decisions.
		Place ADL directives in designated location.

Day 11

TASK	RESPONSIBILITY	ACTIONS
Rehab delivery records forwarded to RNAC	OT, PT, speech, respiratory therapy	RNAC reviews, places information on MDS Section P.
Restorative nursing P3 delivery records evaluated	RNAC	Ensure requirements are met to record for P3 services: care plan delivery records with minimum 15 min/day.

Days 12–13

TASK	RESPONSIBILITY	ACTIONS
MDS hardcopy entered into computer	Data entry	Enter information, check edits. Print computer hard copy, forward to RNAC, who notifies all disciplines that MDS is available for review.

Days 13–14

TASK	RESPONSIBILITY	ACTIONS
Completed MDS reviewed	RNAC, dietary, activities, social services	Review MDS document. If any discrepancies, immediately alert RNAC. Finalize preparation for care conference. Make a worksheet for conference.

Day 14		
TASK	**RESPONSIBILITY**	**ACTIONS**
MDS and RAP summary completed	RNAC Data entry	Double check for accuracy and elimination of errors. Ensure location of information is indicated on RAP summary sheet. Location of information on triggered RAPs will be related to discipline assessment and nursing assessment, or nursing assessment and individual RAP or risk assessment forms. RNAC indicates RAPs that were proceeded on that were not triggered, and where information is located. RNAC signs MDS and notes end date.
Pull Quality Indicators (QIs) Run RUGs score	RNAC Data entry	Give information to RNAC. If unable to run QIs, RNAC uses QI worksheet, takes to care conference.

Days 15–21

TASK	RESPONSIBILITY	ACTIONS
Hold professional care conference per preset schedule	ALL DISCIPLINES	Review and discuss worksheet Discuss core plans developed. Revise, combine, and delete as needed to ensure the most focused plan is developed. Review status of any immediate needs care plans. Can any be eliminated or moved to core plan? Check ADL directives and make any adjustments. Write integrated progress note reflecting proceedings and outcome. DO NOT REPEAT INFORMATION ON THE RAPs or CARE PLAN. REFERENCE IT!
Day 21: Lock MDS for transmission	Social service or team-designated person	Call resident, family into conference. If not in attendance, contact family via phone and/or mail. Discuss plans with resident if possible.
	Data entry	Print verification report. Forward report to designated persons.

Pathway: Quarterly and Significant Change Assessment and Care Plan

There is a 14-day period of assessment and observation for completion of the MDS. Day one of the assessment period begins two weeks to the day PRIOR to the scheduled care conference. During this time, professional reviews are completed and collection of critical data (ADL, mood/behavior tracking, rehab, and restorative service delivery) is completed. The MDS ARD is one week to the day PRIOR to the scheduled conference, with the MDS end date the day preceding the conference. This allows a definite observation period, as well as time for completion of RAP protocols in the event of a significant change.

Example of how time frames are established: If the conference is scheduled on Wednesday the 14th, Wednesday the 1st is day one of the assessment and observation period. Wednesday the 8th is the MDS ARD, and Tuesday the 13th is the MDS end date.

Significant status changes

Transient changes do not require a new MDS assessment. Permanent or major changes—those reflecting a consistent pattern of change (either two or more areas of decline, or two or more areas of improvement)— require a comprehensive assessment, inclusive of RAPs. This must be completed within 14 days of determining the changes exist. If you are unsure of a significant change, after a reasonable period of time, err on the side of completing a new MDS. During the observation period, be sure that problems and needs are identified and addressed on the plan of care.

Once a significant status change has been determined, a new MDS must be initiated. To determine if a significant change has occurred, consider the following non-inclusive guidelines:

1.   Decision-making changes from 0 or 1 to 2 or 3 for item B4 on the MDS

2.   Emergence of sad or anxious mood that is not easily altered

3.   Any decline in an ADL where the resident is newly coded as 3, 4, or 8 for item G1a on the MDS

4.   Incontinence pattern changes from 0 or 1 to 2, 3, or 4, or there is placement of an indwelling catheter

5.   Emergence of unplanned, unexpected weight loss/gain: 5% in 30 days; 10% in 180 days

6. Emergence of pressure ulcers at Stage II or higher, when no ulcers were previously present

7. New use of trunk restraint or chair to prevent rising when not used previously

8. Overall deterioration of condition

9. Emergence of a condition or disease judged to be unstable

Quarterly and significant change assessment procedure

1. All disciplines will complete a quarterly assessment for all routinely scheduled conferences using the designated forms. Significant changes noted as part of a quarterly review are handled in the same manner with the addition of completed "standalone" triggered RAPs.

   The only exception to this is residents evaluated within the previous 30 days who are being cycled into a predetermined conference schedule. In these cases, the MDS will need to be reviewed to ensure no changes have occurred, as well as to establish a new ARD and end date. A review of the recently completed assessments and care plan is also needed, along with a brief progress note reflecting the current status and any modifications to the plan. Professional assessments are to be initiated the week prior to designated ARD. The ARD sets the clock and determines the review period.

   Professional assessments must be completed and placed in the designated location by the ARD to enable the RN responsible for care (RNAC) to consider all data prior to responding to the MDS. While the assessments of dietary, social service, and activities may include part of the MDS look-back period; the primary intent of these assessments is to do a retrospective review and analysis of the previous three months. Data tracking tools completed by nursing for ADLs, mood, and behavior will ensure that the MDS seven-day time-sensitive items are covered for the ARD time requirements. The RN responsible for care will distribute data collection tools to nurses and aides the week preceding the MDS ARD.

2. MDS ARD is EXACTLY one week prior to scheduled conference date. For example, if conference is the third Wednesday of the month, the second Wednesday is the MDS ARD. This means the ADL and mood and behavior trackers would be initiated the first Thursday of the month and completed the second Wednesday.

3. RNAC reviews all professional assessments, tracking tools, and care plan components. These data are assimilated and holistic responses are made to all sections of the MDS within two to five days of the ARD. This allows any remaining time to be used to convert the MDS and complete the RAPs in the event of a significant status change. If a significant change has occurred, only triggered RAPs need to be reviewed. It is not necessary for a discipline to revert to the full comprehensive professional assessment. The review is to be completed using the "standalone" RAP formats on triggered RAPs.

    The MDS will be technically complete at least two days before the scheduled conference. For purposes of computer data entry the official end date will be day 14, the day of conference.

    This enables completion of the RAPs if a significant status change has occurred prior to a scheduled care conference, in keeping with established time frames.

4. All disciplines review the completed MDS in conjunction with their professional assessment and the current care plan PRIOR to the conference. Be prepared to report on status of goals and interventions you are responsible for and to offer input on other problems and needs.

5. At the conference, address all existing care plan goals from the core plan. The note should reflect the status of each goal and team opinion regarding the reason for unmet goals. The team note is to reflect conference proceedings and outcome, inclusive of rationale for care plan additions, modifications and/or continuance of the existing plan. All team members then sign the note, indicating consensus.

Significant status changes occurring outside of quarterly reviews
Procedure

1. RN responsible for care (RNAC) alerts all team members of the change and establishes the ARD for the MDS, then follows the quarterly pathway.

2. All disciplines complete "periodic" professional assessment the weekdays preceding the MDS ARD.

3. RNAC distributes ADL, mood, and behavior tracking tools and fall- and skin-risk RAP assessments week prior to ARD, to ensure data capture is obtained for full seven days preceding the MDS ARD, inclusive of the ARD.

4. RNAC completes the MDS form within two to three days of the assessment reference date.

   – Identify triggered RAPs and alert responsible discipline to complete the triggered standalone RAPs assigned to them.

5. The MDS will be technically completed at least two days BEFORE the scheduled conference. For purposes of computer data entry the official end date will be day 14, the day of conference.

6. All disciplines review the completed MDS, develop a worksheet on contents, including pertinent information from the professional assessment, review the existing care plan, and attend conference prepared to discuss current status and additional care planning needs.

7. At conference, write a team note reflecting the reason for the significant status change, then the proceedings and outcome, inclusive of rationale for care planning additions, modifications and/or continuance of the existing plan. All team members sign the note, indicating consensus.

Quarterly and significant change pathway

Days 1–7		
TASK	**RESPONSIBILITY**	**ACTIONS**

Nursing ADL, mood and behavior tracking	Charge nurse/nurse aide	1. RNAC distributes data collection tools, instructs as needed.
		
		2. CN interviews nursing assistant at end of each shift and completes documents.
		
		   – ADL tracker
		
		   – Mood and behavior tracker

Social service assessment	Social services	1. Review medical record, ADL, immediate needs care plan, core care plan.
		
		2. Talk with resident, family, staff about mood, behavior, well being over the course of the previous three months, particularly occurrences over the previous 30 days.
		
		   – If physical restraints or psychoactive medication is in use, evaluate impact on psychosocial status. Ensure consent forms in place and reflective of what is currently being done.
		
		3. Verify status of advanced care directives, self administration of medication, next of kin addresses and phone numbers.
		
		4. Complete quarterly assessment and analysis.
		
		5. Prepare for care conference:
		
		   - Summarize the resident's course over the previous quarter.
		
		   - Your opinion on the status of care plan goals.
		
		   - Emerging patterns/trends, needs, or problems requiring additional care planning by the team.

Days 1–7 (cont.)

TASK	RESPONSIBILITY	ACTIONS

Activity assessment	Activity staff	1. Review medical record, ADL, immediate needs care plan, core care plan.
		
		2. Talk with staff, resident, and family about time spent pursuing interests, socialization, and time awake and available for interest and activities.
		
		   – Review participation records and areas of involvement over the previous quarter.
		
		   – If physical restraints or psychoactive medications are in use, evaluate influence on activity participation and involvement.
		
		3. Complete quarterly assessment and analysis.
		
		4. Prepare for care conference:
		
		   – Summarize the resident's course over the previous quarter.
		
		   – Describe your opinion on the status of care plan goals.
		
		   – Explain emerging patterns/trends and needs or problems requiring additional care planning by the team.

Dietary assessment	Dietitian or diet tech	1. Review medical record, meds, ADL, immediate need, CORE care planning.
		
		2. Review weight records, intake records, observe resident at meal, interview resident, staff.
		
		   – If the resident receives parenteral or enteral feedings, check that nursing is recording what is actually delivered versus what has been ordered.
		
		3. Complete quarterly assessment and analysis.
		
		4. Prepare for care conference:
		
		   – Summarize the resident's course over the previous quarter.
		
		   – State your opinion on the status of care plan goals.
		
		   – Describe emerging patterns/trends, needs, or problems requiring additional care planning by the team.

Day 8		
TASK	**RESPONSIBILITY**	**ACTIONS**
Forward active therapy delivery records	RNAC gets reports from: • Occupational • Physical • Speech • Respiratory	1. Therapist forwards service delivery minutes for past seven days including the ARD. 2. RNAC ensures treatment order is present, place data in Section P.
Restorative nursing delivery record and program require-ments reviewed	Restorative nurse RNAC	1. Place data in Section P. Note: To claim P3 service there must be care plan with functional problem and measurable goal, delivery records reflecting minimum of 15 min./day, and periodic progress note present from nursing. 2. Progress note reflects status. Indicate future plan for the program. Will it be continued indefinitely? If so give rationale.
All professional assessments completed and on chart	Dietary Social service Activity Other	Place forms in designated area of chart.
MDS is opened on computer	Data entry	MDS is opened.
MDS ARD Begin response to MDS items	RNAC	1. Note the ARD on the MDS form. 2. Begin review of all professional assessments, and data coll-ected. Validate and clarify info as needed. Examine resident. 3. Respond holistically to MDS items.

 The Big Book of Care Plans, Second Edition

Days 11–12

TASK	RESPONSIBILITY	ACTIONS
MDS document completed	RNAC	
Enter MDS into the computer	Data entry	Check for errors, omissions, edits. 1. Print out hard copy, QIs, and RUG scores if applicable. 2. Print hard copy for final review.
Review for significant status change	RNAC	Check for significant status change. If present, alert disciplines to triggered RAPs they are delegated to do. Initiate MDS document changes.

Days 11–13

TASK	RESPONSIBILITY	ACTIONS
If significant change, identify triggered RAPs and begin RAP review	Designated disciplines	Complete "standalone" RAPs. Write analysis and decision on reverse side of form. RNAC indicates location of information on the RAP summary form as the dated RAP (e.g. "1/2/99 Tube Feeding RAP").

Days 12–13

TASK	RESPONSIBILITY	ACTIONS
All disciplines review MDS contents	ALL	1. Review MDS responses, discuss any discrepancies with RNAC.
Continue triggered RAP review if significant change	Designated disciplines	2. Be prepared to discuss POC goals and any changes or additions including rationale for them.
Review care plan in preparation for conference	ALL	
If significant change triggered, RAP review completed and MDS worksheet developed	Designated disciplines	Review care plan for modification or additions related to RAP decisions.
Care plan review and conference preparation completed	ALL	

Day 14

TASK	RESPONSIBILITY	ACTIONS
Care conference	ALL	1. Facilitator presents overview of resident status.
	Designated disciplines	2. Review status of each core plan goal. Make any needed adjustments.
	ALL	3. Review ADL directives; discuss any pattern/trends related to immediate needs care plan occurring through the quarter.
		4. Define any new problems, needs, complications, or risk factors, and care plan accordingly.
		5. Write a team progress note reflecting conference proceedings, as well as action and rationale for unmet goals.
		6. All sign team note and care plan review.
MDS end date entered	RNAC	Date and sign MDS document.
MDS locked for transmission	Data entry	

Annual Assessment Procedure

An annual assessment must always be completed within one year of the last assessment. A comprehensive assessment consists of the MDS and triggered RAP reviews. An annual assessment can always be done before a year passes, but it may not occur later than one year after the previous assessment.

An annual assessment does not necessitate a new plan of care, rather a review of the existing plan for continued accuracy.

1. MDS Assessment Reference Date (ARD) is EXACTLY one week prior to scheduled conference date. For example, if the conference is the third Wednesday of the month, the second Wednesday is the MDS ARD.

    Comprehensive professional assessments incorporating the RAPs are done. All assessments must be completed and on the chart one week prior to conference by the designated MDS ARD, to enable the RN responsible for care (RNAC) to holistically consider all data prior to responding to the MDS items.

    The RN responsible for care (RNAC) will distribute data collection tools to nurses and nurse aides the week preceding the MDS ARD. At a minimum this consists of ADL, mood and behavior tracking tools, and fall- and skin-risk RAP assessments.

2. The RNAC will complete the MDS document within two to three days of the ARD. Identify and begin review of any remaining triggered RAPs.

3. The MDS will be technically completed at least two days BEFORE the scheduled conference. This allows all disciplines to review the MDS and clarify any discrepancies. For purposes of computer data entry the official end date will be day 14, the day of conference.

4. All disciplines are to review the completed MDS, develop a worksheet on contents, including pertinent information from the professional assessment, review the existing care plan, and attend conference prepared to discuss current status and additional care planning needs.

    Note: Should a team member be unable to attend the conference, his or her information and analysis is to be given to another member for presentation.

5. At conference, write a team note reflecting the proceedings and outcome, inclusive of rationale for care planning additions, modifications and/or continuance of the existing plan. All team members sign the note, indicating consensus.

Pathway: Annual assessment

An annual assessment is completed within 12 months of the last full assessment. A comprehensive assessment is defined as completion of the MDS and review of triggered RAPs to determine if care planning is necessary. The annual assessment may be done sooner than 12 months from the last comprehensive assessment, but never later.

There is a defined 14-day period of assessment and observation for completing the Minimum Data Set. The time frame is set based on a selected care conference date. Day one of the assessment begins two weeks to the day PRIOR to care conference. During this time, professional review and collection of pertinent data are completed. The MDS Assessment Reference Date (ARD) is one week to the day PRIOR to scheduled conference, with the MDS completed at least two days before conference. The official "end date" will be the day of conference. This allows a definite observation period, and ample time to complete professional assessments and RAP protocols.

Example of how time frames are established: If conference is scheduled on Wednesday the 14th, Wednesday the 1st is day one of the assessment and observation period, Wednesday the 8th is the MDS start date, and Wednesday the 14th is the MDS end date.

Days 1–7

TASK	RESPONSIBILITY	ACTIONS

ADL tracking
 	
Mood and behavior tracking
	Charge nurse and aide	1. RNAC distributes data collection tools, instructs as needed.
		
		2. CN interviews nursing assistants at end of each shift and completes documents.
		
		   — ADL tracker
		
		   — Mood and behavior tracker

Nursing assessment and RAP review for vision, dental, communication	Charge nurse	RNAC assigns nursing assessment and risk assessments to CNs.

Fall-, skin-risk assessment	RNAC	RNAC evaluates resident and the completed documents for accuracy.
		
		   — Make additional entry on nursing assessment if needed to indicate decisions on vision, dental, and communication RAPs.
		
		   — Review any at risk plans in place, modify as needed.

Day 6 If incontinent — Initiate B&B and I&O tracking sheet	RNAC, charge nurse/nurse aide	RNAC gives tracking tools and instructions to charge nurses. Charge nurses instruct nursing assistants to collect data every two hours for three days. CN reviews results with nursing assistant at end of each shift and ensures they are recorded.
Social service assessment and RAP review for cognition, mood, behavior, well being	Social service	1. Talk with resident, family, staff about mood, behavior, well being over the course of the previous three months, particularly occurrences over the previous 30 days. — If physical restraints or psychoactive medications are used, evaluate impact on psychosocial status. Ensure consent forms are in place and reflective of what is currently being done. 2. Review medical record, ADL directives, immediate needs care plan, core plan. 3. Complete assessment. Use narrative to summarize notable changes over the year.

Days 1–7 (cont.)

TASK	RESPONSIBILITY	ACTIONS
		4. Verify status of advanced care directives, self administration of medication, next of kin addresses and phone numbers.
		5. Prepare for conference presentation.
Activity assessment and RAP review	Activity staff	1. Review medical record, ADL, immediate needs care plan, core care plan.
		2. Talk with staff, resident, and family about interests, socialization and time awake and available for interest/activities. If physical restraints or psychoactive medication is in use, evaluate influence on activity participation and involvement. — Review participation records and areas of involvement over the previous quarter and year.
		3. Complete annual assessment, include any notable differences over the year.
		4. Prepare for conference.
Nutritional assessment and RAP review for nutrition, hydration, tube feeding	Dietitian or diet tech	1. Review medical record, meds, ADL, immediate needs care plan, core care plan.
		2. Review weight records, intake records, observe resident at meal, interview resident, staff. — If receiving parenteral or enteral feedings check that nursing is recording what is actually delivered versus what has been ordered.
		3. Complete annual assessment. Include any notable differences over the year.
		4. Prepare for conference.

Days 1–8

TASK	RESPONSIBILITY	ACTIONS
Restraint RAP, review if used	RNAC	Review RAP, side effects monitor, care plan, and restraint progress notes. Update the progress note reflecting review of these documents and status of care planning decisions. Refer to this note on the RAP summary sheet for location of information.
Review psychoactive medication RAP, if used	RNAC	Review RAP, side effects monitor, behavior tracking forms, care plan, and psychoactive drug progress notes. Update a progress note reflecting review of these documents and status of care planning decisions. Refer to this note on the RAP summary sheet for location of information.
ADL RAP review	RNAC or designated restorative nurse	1. Complete or review previous ADL RAP. Write analysis decision-making statement. 2. Review care plan, adjust if indicated. 3. Ensure delivery records are completed and accurate. 4. Ensure requirements are met to record for P3 services: care plan, delivery records with minimum 15 min./day.

Day 8		
TASK	**RESPONSIBILITY**	**ACTIONS**
All professional assessments completed and on chart ADL, mood and behavior tracking completed	Nursing Dietary Social service Activity Other	Place forms in designated location.
MDS OPENED	Data entry	
MDS ARD	RNAC	Note the reference date on MDS.
Rehab delivery records forwarded to RNAC	Occupational Physical Speech Respiration	RNAC reviews, places information on MDS Section P. RNAC checks that order for therapy services is in place.

Days 8–10		
TASK	**RESPONSIBILITY**	**ACTIONS**
Begin response to MDS items	RNAC	Begin review of all medical records, data collected, and professional assessments. Validate and clarify info as needed.

Day 9		
TASK	**RESPONSIBILITY**	**ACTIONS**
Complete incontinence RAP if indicated	RNAC or designated restorative nurse	1. Review tracking records. 2. Review continence management plan. 3. Complete incontinence RAP or review previous RAP. Write analysis and status of care planning decisions.

Days 10–12

TASK	RESPONSIBILITY	ACTIONS
MDS document completed	RNAC	Forward to data entry.
MDS entered into computer	Data entry	Check for errors, omissions, edits. Print out Quality Indicators and RUG scores if applicable. Print hard copy for final review.
Identify triggered RAPs, reflecting status on RAP summary sheet	RNAC	Review status of RAPs completed by other disciplines. Clarify as needed.

Days 11–13

TASK	RESPONSIBILITY	ACTIONS
All disciplines review MDS contents, develop worksheet	All disciplines	1. Review MDS responses, discuss any disagreement with RNAC. 2. Develop worksheet "grocery list" for conference. Be prepared to discuss changes, additions, etc.
Complete delirium RAP if triggered (all others should have been done by now)	RNAC	Complete the RAP or review the last delirium RAP completed. Write an analysis on the back of the form or attach a trailer note to previously reviewed RAP.

Day 14		
TASK	**RESPONSIBILITY**	**ACTIONS**
RAP summary sheet completed, signed, dated Note end date on MDS and forward for data entry	RNAC	
Care conference	All disciplines	1. Facilitator presents overview of resident status. 2. Review ADL directives; discuss any pattern/trends related to immediate needs care plan occurring through the quarter. 3. Review status of each core plan goal. – Define any new problems, needs, complications, or risk factors. Make any needed adjustments to existing plan. 4. Write a team progress note reflecting conference proceedings, as well as action and rationale for unmet goals. 5. All sign team note and care plan review.
MDS locked for transmission	Data entry	

Medicare PPS Assessment

There are a minimum of five mandated MDS assessments in a typical 100-day Medicare-eligible stay.

Medicare eligibility generally ends when the resident no longer classifies into the RUGs categories of Rehab, Extensive Services Special Care, or Clinically Complex. At this point the MDS completion is based on certification guidelines.

Additional assessments are required for significant status changes. Medicare requires a significant status change assessment to be completed between day 8 and day 10 following the discontinuance of all therapies: OT, PT, and speech. Other significant change assessments may be needed per certification guidelines. Information on these can be located in the MDS training manual. In the interest of time and efficiency, it is preferable to perform additional MDS assessments to coincide with mandated assessments.

Time frames for mandated Medicare PPS assessments

Type of MDS assessment	Assessment reference dates (ARD)	MDS end date	Coverage and payment days
5 + 3 *	Days 1 to 8 *	Comprehensive admission assessment: by 14th day of admission.	1–14
4 + 5 *	Days 11 to 19		15–30
30 + 5	Days 21 to 34		31–60
60 + 5	Days 50 to 64		61–90
90 + 5	Days 80 to 9_ *	All others: by 14th day of ARD	91–100
* Grace days. Days that ARD can be extended without penalty.	* You cannot go past day 92 or you will be out of compliance for quarterly certification requirements.		

The MDS ARD sets the time frames (pathway) for data collection and supporting documentation needed to accurately respond to MDS items. The ARD must be flexible to ensure the best-case-mix score possible for the resident.

Based on the resident's health conditions and treatments, determine the best ARD and count backwards to determine the time frames in which data are to be collected, considered, and evaluated for MDS response.

Medicare PPS Policy and Procedure

1. The ARD determines the look-back period of time to be considered in responding to the MDS items. The reference date will be determined by:

    _____

    Responsible person(s)

2. The five-day assessment will be used to meet certification requirements for a comprehensive assessment (including RAPs) by the 14th day of admission. The day of admission is to be counted as day one of the 14 days. The ARD is to be counted inclusively as the 14th day.

3. Regardless of which ARD is selected for the five-day review (days one through eight), the MDS end date will always be day 14. Other mandated assessment end dates will be up to 14 days from the selected ARD. Determination of the ARD depends on the classification group being sought.

    Rehab classification: ARD will be day five, six, seven, or eight for the five-day assessment (whichever one yields five days of therapy with maximum number of service delivery minutes). The ARD for all other assessments will be based on the five days with the maximum number of service delivery minutes, or, if low rehab category, three days with 45 minutes and two restorative P3 nursing programs six days/week, 15 minutes/day.

Extensive services: **Special care** **Clinically complex**	ARD will be day one through eight for the five-day assessment, dependent on which will capture the most service. It may also be advantageous to use earlier ARDs of the 11th to 13th for the 14-day assessment.
Rationale:	ARD look-back includes some hospital treatments and services.

4. Responses on the MDS will be made using the ARD look-back time period inclusive of transfer and medical records, evaluations, treatment plans, and delivery records occurring in the ARD time periods.

The Big Book of Care Plans, Second Edition

5.   Should a resident be discharged prior to day eight, the MDS will be completed using available information. This may require some judgments and estimates to be made, particularly in the area of ADLs.

6.   Look-back information comes from multiple sources. All of these sources are considered when responding to the MDS items.

7.   Professional assessments for dietary, social services, and activities involve a retrospective and concurrent review of the resident's status. Each discipline is responsible for completing assessments and medical records in the required time frames. For a five-day comprehensive review, these assessments will be completed and in the designated location by day's end on the ARD.

8.   Nursing will track critical data elements of ADLs, mood, and behavior in the ARD period. This tracking will be done continuously through the 30-day ARD. Thereafter they will be initiated in the ARD time period to capture the full seven-day picture on critical items.

9.   The RNAC will review all data and assess the resident, responding holistically to MDS items.

10. Completed MDS will be reviewed by the team for consensus prior to recording end date and locking the MDS.

Medicare Standard Pathway Based on Selected ARD

1. ADL and mood/behavior trackers

   - Initiate on admission day, continue through 30-day ARD

   - All other MDSs: Six days prior to ARD, plus ARD

2. Open the MDS on selected ARD.

3. Notify team of selected date.

4. MDS end dates

   - Five-day assessment is 14th day of admission

   - All other assessments are up to 14th day inclusive of ARD

5. MDS locked seven days from end date

6. For the five-day comprehensive assessment

   Day 1

   - Nursing comprehensive assessment

   - Fall-risk RAP (initiate at-risk POC if indicated)

   - Skin-risk RAP (initiate at-risk POC if indicated)

   - Restraint RAP and analysis prior to accepting or requesting order for use

   - Initiate immediate needs care planning and nurse's notes for CMI/RUG category and other areas of significant concern and need

   Day 1 to 3

   - Psychoactive drug RAP and analysis if in use (initiate protocol).

   - ADL RAP if other than independent. (If seeking low rehab or clinically complex categories, otherwise it may be complete by day 14.)

Day 1 to 5

- Activities, social service, and dietary assessments completed to enable the RNAC to consider the data when responding to the MDS

Three days prior to ARD:

- B&B and I&O tracking for incontinence

RNAC judgment on time frames (no later than day 14)

- Delirium RAPs if symptoms are present

- Incontinence RAP & Initiate Continence Management program

7. The RNAC will respond to all MDS items by day eight. Any remaining RAPs not yet reviewed will be completed by nursing prior to day 14, the MDS end date.

8. Although conferences and meetings regarding the skilled status and Medicare utilization will occur on a frequent basis following admission, the decision for a "Formal Care Conference" will be at the discretion of the team. The team assumes responsibility for ensuring that a comprehensive care plan is in place.

14-Day Assessment: Open MDS on ARD

1. RNAC reviews information from ADL and mood and behavior trackers, immediate needs care plans, and nurse's notes, medication and treatment sheets, and medical record.

2. RNAC collects delivery record information from rehab and restorative nursing.

3. RNAC evaluates resident and interviews family and caregivers as needed.

4. RNAC reviews other disciplines' notes. Discuss resident status as needed with dietary, social services, and activities. If pertinent information to support MDS coding is not in record, make a note at this time summarizing this data.

   • It is not necessary for these disciplines to complete a periodic assessment at this point. You may, however, choose to do so.

5. RNAC assimilates data from all sources. Complete the MDS within two to three days of ARD.

   • Do not sign off or indicate end date at this time. You have up to 14 days from ARD to do this. Waiting buys time to ensure accurate assessment and allows ample time for locking and transmitting.

6. Other disciplines review the completed MDS for consensus.

7. RNAC signs and notes end date on the assessment. Hard copy entered into computer by data entry.

30-, 60-, 90-Day Open MDS on ARD

1. RNAC reviews information from ADL and mood and behavior trackers, immediate needs care plans and nurse's notes, medication and treatment sheets, and medical record.

2. RNAC collects delivery record information from rehab and restorative nursing.

3. RNAC evaluates resident and interviews family and caregivers as needed.

4. Dietary, social service, and activities complete periodic assessment.

5. RNAC assimilates data and responds to MDS items.

6. Each discipline reviews the MDS for consensus and accuracy.

7. RNAC signs and notes end date on the assessment. Hard copy entered into computer by data entry.

MDS Admission Assessment Pathway: All Residents

Admission assessment Medicare 5 day	Use FULL Professional Assessment containing assigned RAPs ⇨ Nursing Assessment (Includes RAPs for Communication, Dental, Vision) ⇨ Social Service (Includes RAPs for Mood, Behavior, Well Being, Cognition) ⇨ Dietary
Professional assessment time frame	Within 1st 24 hours ⇨ Nursing Assessment ⇨ ADL and Mood/Behavior Tracker (Medicare will have continuous use through 30-day ARD) ***Always Nursing RAPS*** ⇨ Skin-Risk RAP ⇨ Fall-Risk RAP ⇨ Restraint RAP if ordered or considering use ***Day 4 to 7*** ⇨ Psychoactive Drug RAP if in use ⇨ B&B tracker x 3 days if Incontinent ⇨ ADL RAP ***Day 1 through 5*** ⇨ Dietary Social Service Activities
Assessment reference date	**Encoder** opens MDS on selected ARD Days _____ **Unit Manager** assimilates data and completes all MDS items
Activities, dietary, social service MDS verification	_____ Days from ARD ❖ Review working copy of the MDS. ❖ Discuss any areas of conflicts (factual or opinion-based) with Unit Manager. ❖ Initial upper-right-hand corner of MDS. ❖ Unit Manager revises if needed and gives to Encoder.
MDS completed	Day _____ TEAM IS NOW FINISHED WITH THE MDS.
Care conference	Days _____ ❖ Care conference held. ❖ Care plan reviewed and finalized.
MDS end date	Day 14 End date added to MDS and RAP summary. All data entered into computer by Encoder. Encoder notes care plan completion date by day 21. Encoder locks within 7 days for transmission. ❖ DELIRIUM RAP, if triggered, is by unit manager by day 14 for annual review.

MDS Quarterly, Significant Change, and Annual Assessment Pathway

Type of assessment	Quarterly ***Social Service, Dietary, Activities*** Use Periodic/Quarterly Assessment Form. If quarterly converts to Significant Change complete standalone RAPs assigned to your discipline IF they trigger Annually ***Social Service, Dietary, Activities, and Nursing*** Use FULL Professional Assessment containing assigned RAPs **Nursing** Full Assessment ⇨ Skin-Risk RAP ⇨ Fall-Risk RAP
Assessment time frames	***Quarterly and Annual*** Within 6 days of assigned ARD (Assessment Reference Date) complete professional assessment. DAY: 1 2 3 4 5 6 up to ARD ***Dietary, Social Service, Activities*** Nursing **initiates ADL and Mood/Behavior Tracker 6 days prior to ARD, plus the ARD date.** On quarterly: *NO specific Nursing Assessment. Episodic Nurses Notes, IMPOCNN, and Monthly Comprehensive Nurses Summary* are used to assimilate data. **On annuals** this info is also used in conjunction with full nursing assessment. *If Quarterly converts to Significant Change, standalone RAPs are completed by the assigned discipline.*
Assessment reference date	***Encoder*** Opens MDS: Day 1 ARD Day 1 (ARD), 2 and 3 Unit Manager assimilates data and completes all MDS items
Activities, dietary, social service MDS verification	***Days 4, 5, 6 from ARD*** ❖ Review working copy of the MDS. ❖ Discuss any areas of conflicts (factual or opinion-based) with Unit Manager. ❖ Initial upper-right-hand corner of MDS. ❖ Unit Manager revises if needed and gives to Encoder.
MDS completed	Day 7 TEAM IS NOW FINISHED WITH THE MDS.
Care conference	Day 8 to 13 Care conference held. Care plan reviewed and finalized.
MDS end date	Day 14 All data entered into computer by Encoder. End date added to MDS and RAP summary (if annual or sig. chg.). Encoder notes care plan completion date by day 21. Encoder locks within 7 days for transmission.

MDS Medicare 14-, 30-, 60-, and 90-Day Assessment Pathway

Type of assessment	**14-Day** ***Social Service, Dietary, Activities*** No specific assessment is needed. Supporting documentation will appear in your progress notes if appropriate. 30-, 60-, 90-*Day ***Social Service, Dietary, Activities*** Use Periodic/Quarterly Assessment Form. * Will use as quarterly if possible.
Assessment time frame	***30-, 60-, 90-*Day*** Within 6 days of assigned ARD (Assessment Reference Date) complete professional assessment. DAY: 1 2 3 4 5 6 up to ARD ***Dietary, Social Service, Activities*** Nursing **initiates ADL and Mood/Behavior Tracker as directed by Unit Manager** *NO specific Nursing Assessment. Episodic Nurses Notes, IMPOCNN, and Weekly/Monthly Comprehensive Nurses Summary* are used to assimilate data. If any assessment converts to Significant Change, standalone RAPs are completed by the **assigned discipline.**
Assessment reference date	***Encoder*** Opens MDS: Day 1 ARD Day 1 (ARD), 2, and 3 Unit Manager assimilates data and completes all MDS items
Activities, dietary, social service MDS verification	***Days 4, 5, 6 from ARD*** ❖ Review working copy of the MDS. ❖ Discuss any areas of conflicts (factual or opinion-based) with Unit Manager. ❖ Initial upper-right-hand corner of MDS. ❖ Unit Manager revises if needed and gives to Encoder.
MDS completed	Day 7 TEAM IS NOW FINISHED WITH THE MDS.
Care conference	Care conferences and care plans are a daily review process by involved team members. Meetings are held with resident and families as needed.
MDS end date 14 days from sARD (including the ARD)	Day 14 All data entered into computer by Encoder. End date added to MDS and RAP summary (if indicated). Encoder locks within 7 days for transmission.

MDS and Care Conference Schedule

Month of _____   Unit _____

Resident name	Room number	Type of assessment	Professional assessments completion window	ARD	IDT MDS consensus window	MDS end date	Care conference date	Comments

Understanding and Documenting RAPs, Clinical Assessments, and Care Conferences

Introduction

The information in this section is designed to provide ideas and alternatives to better assess and develop the residents' plan of care. It presents concepts and approaches to facilitate real interdisciplinary care planning. Interdisciplinary means everyone is looking at the whole person, not just "their part" (that's multidisciplinary!). When everyone sees the individual as multifaceted, the result will be better care that serves the resident and his or her loved ones.

Federal regulatory requirements are consistent throughout the United States. State regulations may impose additional requirements and/or varying interpretations on the intent of the requirements. Be sure you know what is regulation versus what is individual surveyor interpretation. In general regulations dictate what must be done. How it occurs is typically up to the individual facility.

This section has been created to provide the user with the most up-to-date information available at the time of printing. The user assumes full responsibility for use of the section. You are cautioned to stay abreast of regulatory changes and challenged to improve upon the ideas and content from your own experience.

Successful Care Planning

The care planning process begins with professional assessments. Nursing initiates the process at the time of admission, continuing throughout the resident's stay. Shortly after admission social service, dietary, and activities begin their review and evaluation of the residents. These professional assessments lay the groundwork for the comprehensive assessment, which consists of the Minimum Data Set (MDS) and Resident Assessment Protocols (RAPs). Therapy may be involved in the assessment and care planning process from the outset, or may be brought on board as the assessment process unfolds or as residents change.

The MDS

The MDS is a multipurpose functional tool. The MDS lays the foundation for survey, serves as a reimbursement tool for Medicare (and in some states Medicaid), provides valuable data that are converted into Quality Indicators, and, finally, acts as a general quality assurance check on the resident's functional status. The MDS identifies actual and potential problem areas that require further evaluation and investigation. These are referred to as "triggers." These triggers begin the specific analysis—an in-depth review of the related RAP (Resident Assessment Protocol).

Getting the MDS completed

There are different ways to get the MDS completed.

1. Many facilities opt to assign each discipline a section of the MDS to fill out. This is not the ideal method, but it is familiar in a task-oriented model of care planning (which the Resident Assessment Instrument was designed to replace).

    This method typically creates a multidisciplinary approach to resident care rather than an interdisciplinary one. Each discipline completes "its" section, and the MDS Coordinator bears the brunt of the burden as he or she is the only one who has the completed the picture of the resident.

    Typically each discipline only reviews "its" section prior to care conference. While this model appears to share the wealth of work, it actually increases the workload for everybody and creates inaccuracies in the assessment. Each discipline is (or should be) talking to the staff on all three shifts, presumably mindful of the time-sensitive nature of the MDS information. Not only does this create a duplication of work effort and time consumption for the floor staff, it also results in pressure to have each discipline's assessment "match" the MDS, and to have each discipline initiate its assessment on the same date.

2. A more integrated, efficient, and effective approach is to have each discipline complete its pro-fessional assessment PRIOR to the MDS assessment reference date. The assessments should incor-porate MDS items that staff members have knowledge of or need to review. This may mean current assessments need to be revised.

    The MDS coordinator then reviews each discipline's assessment data and completes the MDS using a holistic response. If there were questions or significant variances in data, the coordinator would contact the discipline to clarify the data. In these situations there are two probabilities. The first is that there is a factual error, in which case the records are righted. The second is an opinion-based difference. Opinion-based issues should result in the most agreed-on response being made on the MDS, and an active discussion of the dissenting opinions at care conference (these are true care planning issues).

    In order to keep the MDS timed data up to date and reflective of the assessment time zones, ADL and mood and behavior tracking forms are completed by the direct care staff and nurses in charge. This ensures that any changes in the resident are known and the most accurate response is made on the MDS. If, when reviewing all the data to complete the MDS, the coordinator notes that a discipline is unaware of pertinent facts from the trackers he or she alerts the discipline to the need for an additional progress note. This not only ensures an accurate MDS, but it also acts as a check and balance on communication among and between disciplines.

Important MDS 2.0 Factors

1. **DAY ONE** is the day of admission.

2. The **MDS must be completed** by the 14th day of admission, including the triggered RAPs. All other MDSs must be completed within 14 days of the ARD.

    If the resident is covered by Medicare, two MDSs are required: a five-day and a 14-day. For certification purposes, one of these MDSs serves as the comprehensive assessment inclusive of the RAPs, and MUST be done by the 14th day.

3. **Discharge tracking** form (page 3-2 of the *RAI User's Manual*) must be completed within seven days for ANY healthcare discharge over 24 hours, excluding temporary visits home. Included in this section are items AA 1-7, AB 1-2, A 6, R 3-4, S 10, 11, 12.

__Re-entry tracking__ must be completed within seven days of return for any temporary discharges, when return is anticipated.

4. __Significant Change-in-Status Assessment.__ Look at the WHOLE impact on the resident status. Approximately one in five residents (20%) experiences a decline in status in a six-month period.

   ❑ Not self-limiting

   ❑ Impact on more than one area of health status

   ❑ Care plan requires review or revision

   __Non-significant guidelines__

   ❑ Discrete and easily reversible

   ❑ Short-term acute illness

   ❑ Well established, predictable cyclical pattern

   ❑ Resident continuing to make steady progress

   ❑ Stabilized, but to be discharged

   ❑ End-stage disease

The RAPs

The RAPS result from triggered items on the MDS. The RAPs provide a definitive analysis. They are the essence of the assessment process in terms of evaluating cause-and-effect relationships and what, how, and where to care plan. There are four types of RAP triggers. Determining the type of trigger provides a better perspective on what to look for and how to think about the area under review.

1. __Broad screening__ triggers are designed to identify hard-to-diagnosis problems. These include the delirium and dehydration RAPs.

2. __Rehabilitative potential__ triggers are geared to identify residents who may have rehab potential. Some items trigger because they indicate strengths that can be used to offset and/or assist in working

through problems. The ADL, psychosocial well being and communication, cognitive loss, feeding tubes, and urinary incontinence RAPs are examples of these.

3. **Potential problem** triggers determine if underlying issues are present that increase risk for negative outcomes. Pressure ulcers, feeding tubes, restraints, urinary incontinence, mood, behavior, psychoactive drug, dental, and activity RAPs are examples of these.

4. **Prevention of problem** triggers alert the staff to the presence of risk factors and potential complications. These might include the cognitive loss, mood, behavior, restraints, vision, fall, pressure ulcer, or urinary incontinence RAPs.

The RAPs facilitate decision-making, providing the interdisciplinary team a solid framework for developing the care plan. The structure and content of the care plan are simplified when the team focuses on the assessment process. The assessment includes data collection and data analysis. Without the analysis, time spent collecting information results in a paper-compliant process with care planning that does little to effect positive outcomes for the resident.

In addition to the assessment process, positive outcomes in care planning can be further enhanced with the use of the Quality Indicators. The Indicators are determined by selected responses made on the MDS. The Indicators identify prevalence of certain conditions. When used in conjunction with the resident's plan of care, the Indicators act as a 'crib note' or key to ensure conditions have been appropriately evaluated and care planned. Reviewing the triggered Indicators against the care plan and/or related RAPs to ensure they have been acted on appropriately guarantees your care planning is on target.

Completing the MDS and RAPs

RNAC ROLE: Coordinate, review, respond, and complete the MDS.

Although there are many ways to accomplish completion of the MDS, the method presented in this manual is felt to be the most effective and efficient. Ideally each discipline completes a professional assessment. Each assessment contains MDS items as they relate to a particular discipline. Assessment would be completed PRIOR to the MDS reference date. The RNAC would then review each assessment, including nursing data, and make a holistic response to each item on the MDS. If conflicts were present the RNAC would seek clarification then proceed to make the most appropriate response. Outstanding professional differences would then be discussed at care conference, achieving consensus, if not agreement, on how to proceed.

In this model EACH discipline is responsible for reviewing the completed MDS PRIOR TO CARE CONFERENCE. This eliminates the frequently encountered problems with disciplines only reviewing "their section" of the MDS. This attitude and thought process is the primary culprit for the lack of holistic interdisciplinary care planning and the continued, outdated method of multidisciplinary care planning.

Multidisciplinary care planning demands that each discipline has an assessment and develops a care plan. Disciplines stand alone in this model, distant cousins to one another.

Nursing is the dominant force and so the care plan tends to stay nursing dominated—a surefire way to prevent holistic, interdisciplinary care planning! Multidisciplinary care planning is out. Interdisciplinary care planning or trans-disciplinary care planning is in! The interdisciplinary model demands that each discipline evaluate the resident to determine if it can provide assistance in any way to ensure the best outcome. This model provides support to all disciplines. The most dominant discipline is the one having the greatest ownership/relationship to the problem under review. Disciplines are interdependent (not co-dependent), on one another. They are more like immediate family and next of kin.

Nursing MDS Supporting Documentation

Supporting documents	Who does them	Initiated	Completed
ADL day tracker **Mood and behavior tracker**	Nurse aide provides information. Charge nurse completes form.	Seven days PRIOR to MDS ARD at the end of each shift. • For Medicare PPS complete daily for first 30 days on Medicare-eligible residents.	Data must include day of the MDS ARD. Info can be recorded beginning day 8 on the MDS.
Comprehensive nursing summary	Licensed nurse in conjunction with nurse aide.	Can be weekly or monthly.	As assigned. Reviewed to assist in MDS coding to support responses evaluating status changes from one MDS review period to the next.
Immediate needs care plans and nurse's notes	Predominantly licensed nurses. May also be done by other disciplines.	On identification of acute problem or need requiring routine monitoring or oversight.	As problem needs are resolved and/or no longer require routine monitoring. Ensures accurate MDS coding, particularly related to timed items such as UTIs, fevers, pneumonia, etc.

Dietary MDS Supporting Documentation

*Enables five-day assessment to be used as comprehensive MDS, allowing grace-day use on 14-day assessment.

Supporting documentation	Who does it	Initiated	Completed
Dietary Comprehensive assessment and RAP review for nutrition, hydration, tube feeding	Dietitian	At or shortly after admission. Annually. • For Medicare PPS within the first 5 days of admission.*	No later than MDS ARD. Info will be used to assist in holistic completion of the MDS. Nutrition, hydration, tube-feeding RAPs, and analysis for care planning decisions are located on this document. Location of information on the RAP summary sheet will be this dated assessment for RAPs triggered by MDS.
Dietary Periodic and quarterly assessment	Dietary	The week PRIOR to MDS ARD on all quarterly reviews AND PPS-mandated assessments.	No later than MDS ARD.
Standalone RAPs for nutrition, hydration, tube feeding	Dietary	Significant status change reviews if triggered on the MDS.	No later than MDS end date.
Intake records for parenteral and enteral feedings usually recorded on med/TX record.	Licensed nurse	With use. Reviewed by dietitian in conjunction with completion of dietary assessment.	When discontinued.

Social Services MDS Supporting Documentation

*Enables five-day assessment to be used as comprehensive MDS, allowing grace-day use on 14-day assessment.

Supporting documentation	Who does it	Initiated	Completed
Social service Comprehensive assessment and RAP review for cognition, mood, behavior, and well being	**Social service**	At or shortly after admission. Annually. • For Medicare PPS complete within first 5 days of admission.*	No later than MDS ARD. Info will be used to assist in holistic completion of the MDS. Cognition, mood, behavior, and well being RAPs and analysis for care planning decisions are located on this document. Location of information on the RAP summary sheet will be this dated assessment for RAPs triggered by MDS.
Social service Periodic and quarterly assessment	Social service	The week PRIOR to MDS ARD on all quarterly reviews AND PPS-mandated assessments.	No later than MDS ARD.
Stand alone RAPs for cognition, mood, behavior, well being	Social service	Significant status change reviews if triggered on the MDS.	No later than MDS end date.

© 2009 HCPro, Inc.

Activities MDS Supporting Documentation

*Enables five-day assessment to be used as comprehensive MDS, allowing grace-day use on 14-day assessment.

Supporting documentation	Who does it	Initiated	Completed
Activities Comprehensive assessment activities and RAP review	Activities	At or shortly after admission. Annually. • For Medicare PPS complete within first 5 days of admission.*	No later than MDS ARD. Info will be used to assist in holistic completion of the MDS. Activity RAP and analysis of care planning decision is located on this document. Location of information on RAP summary sheet will be this dated assessment of Activity RAP triggers on MDS.
Activities Periodic and quarterly assessment	Activities	The week PRIOR to MDS ARD on all quarterly reviews AND PPS-mandated assessments.	No later than MDS ARD.
Stand alone RAP for activities	Activities	Significant status change reviews if triggered on the MDS.	No later than MDS end date.

Rehab Therapy MDS Supporting Documentation

Supporting documentation	Who does it	Initiated	Completed
Order for OT, PT, speech evaluation	Therapist via physician order.	Day of order, but no later than 48 to 72 hours after receiving order.	To capture maximum in therapy category 5 days of service must be given during MDS ARD time frames.
Order for treatment (Recommend including modality, frequency, and duration of each session)	Therapist request, nursing ensures transmitted and approved by physician.	For Medicare PPS date treatment initiated needs to be considered in establishing MDS Assessment Reference Date.	When therapy discontinued.
Plan of treatment Must include functional problem, reasonable measurable goal, modalities, and frequency of service, expected duration of therapy.	Therapist providing service. Therapist records based on minutes actually spent treating resident.	On initiation of treatment. On initiation of treatment.	On completion of each service delivered.
Delivery records			RN assessment coordinator records information on the MDS after reviewing minutes of delivery for the 6 days preceding MDS ARD and services provided on the reference date.
Progress notes	Therapist	Per therapy standards.	**Per therapy standards.** Information not needed for MDS but may be invaluable in an exception audit to support therapist activity.

Restorative Nursing Programs MDS Supporting Documentation

Supporting documentation	Who does it	Initiated	Completed
ADL RAP	Assigned nurse. Therapist may be consulted but this is a nursing activity.	Before or when triggered by the MDS. If resident requires staff support, programming must be considered to improve/maintain status, slow decline, or minimize complications.	Within 14 days of MDS ARD if triggered.
Plan of care Identifies functional problem, measurable goal, interventions to meet goal(s) and frequency of service (minutes and days), and service provider. • Must be nursing supervised to qualify for restorative nursing program on the MDS 2.0.	Designated licensed nurse.	As need is identified.	When plan is discontinued.
Delivery records Reflect minutes of service.	Service provider specially trained to carry out the service.	Per plan of care.	Immediately following the delivery of service. RN assessment coordinator records information on the MDS after reviewing minutes of delivery for the 6 days preceding MDS ARD and services provided on the reference date.
Progress notes	Licensed nurse supervising the program.	Per policy.	Per policy.

RAP data collection and data analysis

Data collection and data analysis are the key elements in a resident assessment and care plan. Collecting information is step one. That information is typically placed on a form. Unfortunately, all too often the team sees this as an end product. It is not. Analyzing the information, thinking critically about what it means, determining cause-and-effect relationships is the essence of the process. Reviewing a resident critically is always a team effort and responsibility. Different viewpoints and perspectives ensure the best possible plan.

Assigning RAPs to disciplines is a good idea. The discipline that "seems" closest to the RAP can collect the data and make the initial decision to proceed to care planning. The team retains the right and responsibility to alter the initial decision if additional information indicates a need for a change from the original decision. This change can be documented in a team note. It would not be necessary for the discipline to go back and modify the note. The RAP summary sheet would note location of information at both/all sources.

In order to efficiently and effectively respond to the MDS and collect and analyze data professional assessment tools need to complement and support one another and prevent double work and effort. Assessment/RAP tasks are designed in this format to be done in the following manner:

Assessment Assignments

Dietary assessment	Activity assessment	Social service assessment
Contains RAPs for nutrition, hydration, tube feeding.	Contains RAP for activity.	Contains RAPs for cognition, mood, behavior, well being.
Additional assessments may be needed such as calorie counts, additional lab work, etc.	Additional assessment may be needed such as behavior mapping.	Additional assessments may be needed such as the Global Deterioration Scale, the Geri-Depression Scale, etc.

Nursing assessment

Contains RAPs for vision, communication, and dental.
Completion of the information reflects if additional actions and/or care planning is or is not indicated.

Other outstanding RAPs that trigger on the MDS can be anticipated prior to completing the MDS. These can be done as they are noted or following MDS completion.

- **Physical restraints RAP.** If being considered or ordered MUST have evaluation PRIOR to implementing. The restraint RAP in the Documentation manual serves this purpose well.

- **Psychoactive drug RAP.** If ordered, review is indicated. This RAP can ensure appropriate use in accordance with federal guidelines and establish a baseline for evaluating side effects.

- **ADL RAP.** If other than independent in ADL this RAP will trigger. The indications are for restorative nursing at a minimum and possibly therapy. The RAP can aid in determining the type of care needed—either supportive/maintenance or enhancement/improvement.

- **Delirium RAP.** This RAP triggers easily. It is a broad screening RAP. Review can pick up the need for additional actions to reverse the condition before it becomes a chronic subacute problem.

- **Skin and fall RAPs** are considered in this manual as "always" RAPs. Residents need to be evaluated for presence of risk. Use of guidelines in a numeric format can ensure risk is noted promptly. Floor nurse completes the numeric evaluation. Should the MDS trigger either RAP, the RNAC can choose to pull together the pertinent factors in a narrative summary, including what MDS items prompted the triggering, on the back of the numeric risk assessment.

- **Incontinence RAP.** If any incontinence is present this RAP will trigger. Using the RAP guidelines, along with short-term tracking of in-take and output and elimination habits, provides the information you need to develop an appropriate continence management program.

Analyzing the data to produce meaningful information for care planning

MDS principle
❖ Not all information applies to every resident
❖ All sections of the MDS have value for each discipline
❖ Each discipline must review the completed MDS to be an equal partner on the team
❖ Failure of any professional team member to review the completed MDS prior to care conference does a disservice to everybody

How to get the best results with the MDS 2.0

Develop an MDS 2.0 worksheet. It will provide the pertinent data that need to be considered for care planning. It is the grocery store for care planning. Each discipline can develop its own worksheet, or one worksheet can be developed by the RNAC and copies provided to each discipline PRIOR to conference. Each discipline can then review and, if need be, rearrange the information as they see fit, adding additional data from their professional assessment. This provides everyone with all relevant data collected on the MDS and provides a visual display of how each "aisle"/area relates to the other.

Aisle 1	Diagnosis
Aisle 2	Triggered RAPs
Aisle 3	Problem items
Aisle 4	Strengths/considerations
Aisle 5	Triggered Quality Indicators

MDS Worksheet

Resident name _____ **Date** _____

Directions: List diagnosis from MDS Section I, list RAPs along with note as to why triggered, other problems noted on MDS and your professional assessment, along with strengths identified by MDS and your assessment, then the QIs triggered. Look for the relationships among these items. This will assist you in identifying the care planning problems and needs, and organize your focus for care conference.

Diagnosis	Triggered RAPs	Problem items/ considerations	Strengths	Triggered Quality Indicators

Problems and needs for care planning

_____

_____

_____

_____

_____

_____

_____

_____

_____

_____

_____

RAP principle

❖ No RAP has been reviewed without considering the guidelines contained in the RAP

❖ Collecting and recording data is the beginning of RAP review

❖ RAP review is completed when information has been analyzed and care planning decisions validated

The 18 resident assessment protocols

Delirium	Activities
Cognitive Loss	Falls
Visual Function	Nutritional Status
Communication	Feeding Tubes
ADL Function	Dehydration/Fluid Maintenance
Urinary Incontinence/Catheters	Oral/Dental Care
Psychosocial Well Being	Pressure Ulcers
Mood	Psychotropic Drugs
Behavioral Symptoms	Physical Restraints

How to get the best results with RAPs

There is no mandated method. The facility needs to consider the best options for its circumstances. Here are some recommendations for "best" results and greatest efficiency of data collection:

- Combine RAP guidelines in professional assessments. It is possible to capture 11 RAPs in this manner. You get a more comprehensive assessment and avoid duplication of effort if the RAPs trigger. On the RAP summary sheet indicate location of information as the professional assessment(s).

- Use risk-assessment tools for specific problem-prevention RAPs. Consider Fall- and Skin-Risk assessments as "always" RAPs.

- Complete RAPs as they become evident, particularly those that can create negative outcomes and regulatory headaches. These include Restraints, Psychoactive drugs, and Incontinence.

- The ADL RAP will always trigger unless the person is independent. The sooner you evaluate, the better the outcome and potential impact on case-mix scores.

Understanding the RAPs

The RAPs read like a magazine article. It is important that all professional staff members are acquainted with the content of each RAP. Having a general understanding of what the RAPs are and how they work is an important starting point for all team members.

HOW TO ACCOMPLISH THIS:

MAKE RAPs REQUIRED READING FOR ALL PROFESSIONAL AND LICENSED STAFF.

INCLUDE RAP TRAINING IN ORIENTATION.

The RAPs are divided into four sections.

The first section looks at the general problem area and how it affects the nursing home population. It often provides the focus or objectives of the protocols. This information gives focus and direction to the care plan when decisions to proceed are made.

The second section lists the MDS items that will trigger the RAP review. The trigger indicates a need to evaluate the condition further. "Evaluate" does not mean to proceed automatically to care planning. It means look further, assess to see if there are strengths to work with, real problems, potential problems, and/or rehab capability. The review assists in determining cause-and-effect relationships. Knowing the reason the RAP triggered gives valuable clues. Some RAPs are causative, some may be curative; others will be outcomes of other problems, and some may turn out to be of no consequence.

The third section is the "guts". This is where all factors are considered that cause, contribute to, or exacerbate the triggered condition. Here you consider the data to determine what the playing factors and potential resources are, or where you determine that there is no problem or need for care planning.

The fourth section repeats the triggering items and provides an outline of the information covered in the guidelines. It is a handy reference but does not take the place of reviewing the guidelines.

> It is important to distinguish the difference between having a general knowledge of the Resident Assessment Protocols content and applying the specific application of the guidelines for an individual.

The RAPs provide a holistic perspective for the area under review. Situation dependent, cause-and-effect relationships change. While not mandated, the use of a structured format to review and analyze the guidelines is strongly recommended. This enables close scrutiny of all the playing factors. Combined with the knowledge gained from the MDS and professional assessments a solid foundation will be in place to make the best care planning decisions.

Analyzing the RAPs - KI-S Them!

Determine the key issues (KI) and strengths (S) that apply to the guidelines for the specific resident. After you have collected the data, review the information and identify the key issues and strengths by placing a KI or S next to pertinent items.

This process and those noted items, coupled with the reasons the RAP triggered, are the essence of your analysis and decision-making.

Completing this exercise focuses you on the relevant guidelines that are important for that resident. This is the MOST IMPORTANT part of the process.

Avoid just regurgitating known information...analyze it!

Pre- and Post-Tests

Before you can effectively understand the process and how to analyze RAPs it is very helpful to ensure all your clinical staff understand the RAPs. Make them required reading and give pre- and post-tests to validate the action.

Pre-/Post-Test: Delirium RAP

Each answer counts as 10 points.

1. What is delirium? _____

2. List the four primary characteristics of delirium.

    1. _____
    2. _____
    3. _____
    4. _____

3. The key question when evaluating delirium:

    _____?

4. Assessment steps involve ruling out causes beginning with acute medical problems and drug toxicity. Psychosocial problems and sensory problems must then be evaluated. Identify three of four medication-related problems to be considered as potential culprits.

    1. _____
    2. _____
    3. _____

5. Psychosocial causes can be due to restraint use, relocation, depression, isolation, and _____

Answer key:

1. An acute confusion state that is reversible.

2. 1) fluctuating states of consciousness; 2) disorientation; 3) decreased environmental awareness; 4) behavior changes.

3. Is there a reversible cause?

4. 1) med error; 2) number of meds; 3) meds alone or in combination; 4) new med relationship to symptoms.

5. Recent loss.

 The Big Book of Care Plans, Second Edition

Pre-/Post-Test: Cognitive Loss RAP

Each answer counts as 10 points.

1. **Define cognition.** _____

2. **Cognitive impairment is based on degree of loss in three areas.**

   1. _____
   2. _____
   3. _____

3. **Residents with cognitive loss need to be involved in group activities.**

   a. True   False

   b. Explain rationale for your response.

   _____
   _____

4. **There is a strong relationship between cognitive loss and behavior problems. This is characterized by a catastrophic reaction. What causes this response?**

   _____

5. **There are three primary care planning goals for the cognitively impaired person. List them.**

   1. _____
   2. _____
   3. _____

Answer key:

1. The ability to think in order to know the world.
2. Memory, recall, decision-making.
3. A or b depending on rationale. True if it does not overtax them, false if it does.
4. The person decompensates and acts out.
5. Maintain dignity, preserve functional status/minimize decline, and provide positive experiences that are not overly demanding; lay foundations for reasonable expectation concerning resident abilities and needs, define appropriate support roles for staff.

Pre-/Post-Test: Visual Function RAP

Each answer counts as 10 points.

1. The aged eye requires how much more light to see than the young eye? _____

2. The four leading causes of visual impairment in the elderly are:

   1. _____
   2. _____
   3. _____
   4. _____

3. List at least three consequences of visual loss.

   1. _____
   2. _____
   3. _____

4. The two primary purposes of this RAP are:

   1. _____
   2. _____

Answer key:

1. Three to four times.

2. Macular degeneration, glaucoma, cataracts, diabetic retinopathy.

3. Visual safety, self image problems, reduced participation in social, personal, self-care activities.

4. Identify treatable conditions placing resident at risk for blindness; identify visual problems where resident can be understood and understand; identify vision impairments when the resident cannot be understood or understand; identify visual impairments that could be improved with visual appliances.

The Big Book of Care Plans, Second Edition

Pre-/Post-Test: Communication RAP

Each answer counts as 10 points.

1. Name three benefits of good communication for the resident.

   1. _____

   2. _____

   3. _____

2. Deficits can be wide ranging. Problems can occur with expression or reception or both. List three examples of each of these difficulties.

   Expressive difficulties (i.e. speech and voice production problems)

   1. _____

   2. _____

   3. _____

   Receptive difficulties (i.e. interpreting facial expressions)

   1. _____

   2. _____

   3. _____

3. The key focus of care planning is the consideration of resident strengths and weaknesses related to understanding, hearing, and

   _____

Answer key:

1. Enables resident to express emotion, listen to others, share information, ease adjustment to a strange environment; lessens social isolation and depression.

2. Expressive: finding appropriate words, relaying coherent statements, describing objects and events, gestures and writing. Receptive: difficulty in hearing, speech discrimination in quiet and noisy situations; vocabulary comprehension, vision and reading comprehension.

3. Expression.

Pre-/Post-Test: ADL Functional/Rehabilitation Potential RAP

Each answer counts as 10 points.

1. The MDS triggers two types of resident for ADL RAP review. Name them.

   1. _____

   2. _____

2. Identify three of the four complications of inactivity.

   1. _____

   2. _____

   3. _____

3. The key factor in determining rehab ability is _____

4. The key factor in the success of rehab is resident _____

5. List three of the seven types of rehab goals.

   1. _____

   2. _____

   3. _____

Answer key:

1. Rehabilitation, maintenance/complication avoidance.

2. Pressure ulcers, falls, contractures, muscle wasting, and incontinence.

3. Ability to learn.

4. Motivation.

5. Restore function to maximum self-sufficiency; replace hands on assist with task segmentation or verbal cueing; restore ability to allow to function with fewer supports; shorten time required to provide assist; expand amount of space in which self-sufficiency can be practiced; avoid or delay loss of additional independence; support the resident certain to decline to lessen likelihood of complications.

The Big Book of Care Plans, Second Edition

Pre-/Post-Test: Urinary Incontinence and Indwelling Catheters

Each answer counts as 10 points.

1. **The three primary purposes of this RAP are to**

    1. _____
    2. _____
    3. _____

2. **Identify five of the eight factors necessary for continence.**

    1. _____
    2. _____
    3. _____
    4. _____
    5. _____

3. **List two of the four MOST COMMON causes of reversible incontinence.**

    1. _____
    2. _____

Answer key:

1. Identify reversible causes, improve bladder function, and improve overall quality of life.

2. Bladder that can store and expel, urethra that can open and close right, locomotion (able to reach toilet in time), dexterity (able to adjust/manipulate clothing), cognitive function and social awareness, motivation (resident and staff), fluid balance, integrity of the spinal cord and peripheral nerves.

3. UTI, fecal impaction, delirium, lack of toilet access.

Experiential Learning: Adapted Psychosocial Well Being RAP

Directions: Identify something in your life that is a stressor, creating discomfort, anxiety, concern, or worry. It can be something related to work or home. Think about the FEELINGS this is creating for you. Then respond to each of the items listed below. Following completion, determine the key issues and strengths based on the information you have recorded. On the reverse side, validate whether you need to proceed to action or not.

	Yes	No	N/A	Clarifying information
Were mood or behavior problems present before reduced sense of well being?				
Do mood or behavior problems impact on sense of well being?				
Have previous or current interventions/things you have tried helped with this?				

	Yes	No	N/A	Clarifying information
Have key social relationships been terminated or altered (e.g. loss of family, friends, or others)?				
Have external factors impacted on your well being (e.g., use of a move, certain rules or restrictions, etc.)?				
Does your knowledge or communication style or lack of interest impede interaction with others?				
Are you uncomfortable with other people or in social/group settings?				
Was life more satisfactory before this issue/area/problem came up?				
Are you preoccupied with the past or unwilling to acknowledge/deal with the present situation?				
Do you perceive this to be a serious problem? Do others?				
Are corrective strategies now in use?				
Is this an area that might be improved?				

Experiential Learning: Adapted Psychosocial Well Being RAP (cont.)

Triggering item(s)/reason/prompt for picking this area/issue/problem?

Analysis for needed action

KEY ISSUES

_____

_____

_____

_____

_____

STRENGTHS

_____

_____

_____

_____

_____

HOLD BACKS/RISK FACTORS/POTENTIAL COMPLICATIONS

_____

_____

_____

_____

_____

Decision: ❏ Proceed   ❏ Do not Proceed

Potential for improvement: ❏ Able to be resolved   ❏ Maintain as is   ❏ Minimize/Prevent Complications

Referrals/Contacts Indicated

_____

_____

_____

_____

_____

Pre-/Post-Test: Mood State RAP

Each answer counts as 10 points.

1. Approximately what percentage of nursing home residents have major depression? _____

2. What percentage will exhibit symptoms of a mood-state problem? _____

3. List the four main categories from the MDS that indicate potential mood problems.

    1. _____

    2. _____

    3. _____

    4. _____

4. Passive residents with distressed mood may be overlooked and thought not to have any mood problems. List one potential indicator that may indicate a distressed mood is present for the passive resident.

    _____

5. Mood problems that are not easily altered usually will require two types of therapeutic interventions. Name them.

    _____

    _____

6. Moods that are not easily altered even after initiation of drug therapy indicate additional action is needed. What is it?

    _____

    _____

Answer key:

1. 15%

2. 30%

3. Verbal expressions of distress, sleep cycle issues, sad/apathetic appearance, loss of interest.

4. Shows little/no initiative; remains uninvolved in activities.

5. Antidepressant drug therapy, psychosocial counseling.

6. Review of medication. Length of time receiving, dosage, consideration of different drug.

Pre-/Post-Test: Behavioral Symptoms RAP

Each answer counts as 10 points.

1. What percentage of nursing home residents exhibit behavior problems? _____

2. Over 80% of residents with behavior problems have a deficit in a particular area of function. Name it.

   _____

3. There are five primary categories of behavior symptoms. List three.

   1. _____
   2. _____
   3. _____

4. When behavior is distressing and non-medical interventions have failed, what is the next course of action to be considered?

   _____

5. Most behavior problems that a resident exhibits are out of control of the staff.

   True   False

6. A key factor in determining the need for intervention is

   _____

7. Identify two reasons residents have behavior problems that the staff could lessen or minimize occurrence of.

   _____

   _____

Answer key:

1. 60% to 70%.
2. Cognition.
3. Wandering, verbal abuse, physical abuse, socially inappropriate behavior, resist care.
4. Use of medication.
5. False.
6. Impact on functional status, symptoms causing distress to resident, placing others at risk.
7. Overstimulation, loss of control, lack of comprehension, inability to remember.

Pre-/Post-Test: Activities RAP

Each answer counts as 10 points.

1. **The activity RAP focuses on cases where the system may have failed the resident.**

    True   False

2. **The two possible reasons this RAP will trigger:**

    _____

    _____

3. **List five factors that may hinder resident involvement in activities.**

    _____

    _____

    _____

    _____

4. **List two of five problems to be considered as the activity plan is developed.**

    _____

    _____

Answer key:

1. True.

2. Revise the plan (little to no involvement, prefers change in routine); review the plan (awake all/most of time, involved in most activities).

3. Congestion, toilet access, lighting, location, amount of stimulation present, boredom, depression, shyness, doesn't like activity offered, facility rules.

4. Cognitive status, unstable/acute health conditions, number of treatments received, time in facility, use of psychoactive meds/restraints.

Pre-/Post-Test: Falls RAP

Each answer counts as 10 points.

1. What percentage of nursing home residents fall each year? _____

2. What percentage of these result in fractures or soft tissue injuries? _____

3. Identify the two primary internal (coming from the resident) risk factors.

    1. _____

    2. _____

4. Identify the three broad categories of external risk factors that place the resident at risk.

    1. _____

    2. _____

    3. _____

5. What are the two primary concerns related to falls and psychoactive medications?

    1. _____

    2. _____

Answer key:

1. 40%.

2. 5%/15% = 20%.

3. Physical health, functional status.

4. Medication side effects, use of appliances and restraints, environmental conditions.

5. Orthostatic hypotension, altered sensorium.

Pre-/Post-Test: Nutritional Status RAP

Each answer counts as 10 points.

1. **Hunger is inconsistent with a good quality of life.**

    True   False

2. **An overly managed diet may cause malnutrition.**

    True   False

3. **Fear of eating and drinking may be caused by COPD.**

    True   False

4. **Malnutrition due to poor communication usually indicates substandard care.**

    True   False

5. **List four problems that may impede ability to consume food.**

    1. _____
    2. _____
    3. _____
    4. _____

6. **List two MDS items that trigger a review of this RAP.**

    1. _____
    2. _____

Answer key:

1. True.

2. True.

3. True.

4. True.

5. Chewing problems, swallowing problems, reduced ability to feed self, medical causes.

6. Weight loss, 25% uneaten, ulcers, mech. altered diet, IVs, hunger, taste alterations, nutritional deficiencies.

Pre-/Post-Test: Feeding Tube RAP

Each answer counts as 20 points.

1. **The ONLY rationale for use of tube feedings is**

   _____

2. **Factors that impede removal of tubes**

   1. _____
   2. _____
   3. _____
   4. _____

Answer key:

1. Demonstrated medical needs to prevent malnutrition or dehydration.

2. Comatose, failure to eat AND resist eating, diagnosis of CVA, gastric ulcer, gastric bleeding, chewing problems, swallowing problems, length of time tube has been in place.

Pre-/Post-Test: Dehydration/Fluid Maintenance RAP

#1 and #2 count as 20 points, #3 counts as 10 points.

1. Define dehydration.

   _____

   _____

2. The most crucial symptoms of dehydration are difficult to identify in the aged.

   True   False

3. Identify six of eight signs and symptoms of dehydration.

   1. _____

   2. _____

   3. _____

   4. _____

   5. _____

   6. _____

Answer key:

1. A condition in which fluid loss far exceeds fluid intake.

2. True.

3. Dizziness on sitting/standing, falls, confusion/change in mental status, decreased fluid output, decreased fluid skin turgor/dry mucous membranes, constipation/impaction, fever/infection, decreased functional ability, fluid/electrolyte imbalance.

Pre-/Post-Test: Dental Care RAP

Each answer counts as 20 points.

1. **Having healthy teeth and dentures is important to nutritional adequacy.**

    True   False

2. **Condition of teeth can affect social interaction among residents.**

    True   False

3. **Name two of the three problems that place residents at greatest risk for poor oral health.**

    1. _____

    2. _____

Answer key:

1. True.

2. True.

3. Multiple medical conditions and medications, functional limitations in self care, communication deficits.

Pre-/Post-Test: Pressure Ulcers RAP

Each answer counts as 20 points.

1. What percentage of residents are at risk for developing pressure ulcers? _____

2. Pressure ulcers are one of the most common, preventable conditions in the elderly.

   True   False

3. There are two primary assessment goals. Name them.

   1. _____

   2. _____

4. Other than bedfast/mobility problems and incontinence, identify one other factor placing resident at risk.

   _____

Answer key:

1. 60%.

2. True.

3. Ensure treatment plan is in place with residents with pressure ulcers, to identify at-risk residents not currently receiving some type of program.

4. PVD, previous history of ulcers, skin desensitized to pain or pressure, daily trunk restraint.

Pre-/Post-Test: Psychotropic Drugs RAP

Answer counts on # 1 to 3 as 10 points, #4 is 20 points.

1. **What is the two-part goal of drug therapy?**

    1. _____
    2. _____

2. **List two major side effects of use.**

    1. _____
    2. _____

3. **When evaluating the need for the drug the pros and cons of potential side effects in relation to the amount of distress must be considered. What two other factors must be considered?**

    1. _____
    2. _____

4. **The two prime directives when initiating drug therapy are**

    1. _____
    2. _____

Answer key:

1. Maximize function, minimize side effects.
2. Hypotension, delirium.
3. Amount and type of distress, response to non-pharmacological interventions.
4. Start low, go slow.

Pre-/Post-Test: Physical Restraints RAP

Each Answer counts as 20 points.

1. Use of physical restraints undercuts the major goals of long-term care.

    True   False

2. Use of restraints demands what kind of need be present?

    _____

3. In considering the use of physical restraints the key question to ask is

    _____

4. The one fact you can count on with the use of a physical restraint is

    _____

5. Preventing falls for safety is an acceptable reason for restraint use.

    True   False

Answer key:

1. True.
2. Medical.

3. Why do you want to use it? What do you hope to accomplish?
4. Increased dependence.
5. False.

The Big Book of Care Plans, Second Edition

What Is a Care Conference?

Care conferences are both formal and informal. Informal conferences occur each time resident care or needs are discussed. These conferences occur with various staff members, the resident, and family. Dependent on the nature of the conference, supporting documentation may or may not be indicated. Formal conferences are more structured. They generally involve more than two people and are preplanned. The focus is on care planning needs caused by a significant problem, or in response to assessments completed at regular intervals throughout the year.

Suggested types of conferences

"Getting to know you" conference

Held: First week of admission, 15 to 30 minutes.

Attendance: Social worker, RN responsible for care, resident, family, significant other

Purpose:

- To identify major concerns, fears, and goals of resident and family

- To identify the facility liaison for the resident and family

Example of meeting contents: Do you have particular worries about being here? Do you have a certain routine that you follow?

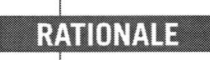 **RATIONALE** Often the first few weeks of admission set the tone for the entire length of stay. Knowing the fears and concerns up front can go a long way to preventing them from materializing. Putting a name to a face provides additional comfort and security.

PPS conference

PPS requires MDS assessments at day 5, 14, 30, 60, and 90. Additionally the determination of a significant status change is expanded under PPS to include a change in case-mix grouping. This does not necessarily mean that a sit-down conference is needed for each review. However, it is imperative that all parties responsible for care delivery are on track and in agreement with the plan, resident status and progress, and the best MDS data capture date.

At a minimum, the following items need to be discussed and considered in the PPS environment.

1. Identifying the best window of opportunity to establish the case-mix score. This means reviewing care and services, and determining the BEST MDS reference date to capture the highest case-mix score. This may mean establishing a reference date earlier or later than typically might be done for a non-Medicare recipient.

2. Ensuring all assessments and tracking tools support the items coded on the MDS.

3. Reviewing critical pathways to ensure care and expected outcomes are on target, and that exceptions are clearly documented and demonstrated to be unavoidable. (Always take a continuous quality improvement, proactive approach: Can we do better?)

4. Evaluating financial and support systems discharge status and discharge planning needs.

Admission conference

Held: 14 to 21 days after admission

Attendance: RN responsible for care, social services, activities, and dietary. Others as needed.

- Resident/family/direct care staff may or may not attend dependent on how facility gains involvement of those with resident care.

- Refer to "Care Conference Attendance Involvement" for a detailed discussion of this topic.

Purpose:

- To complete the care plan following professional assessments, Minimum Data Set, and review of triggered resident assessment protocols

- To ensure that the interdisciplinary team agrees with the MDS and RAP decisions

> **RATIONALE** The interdisciplinary team ensures that a holistic care plan is developed. As a team, the problem and needs of the resident are discussed from the viewpoint of each discipline.

 The Big Book of Care Plans, Second Edition

Content of the meeting:

1. Overview of the resident: where admitted from, general findings of the MDS, adjustment to the facility.

2. Each discipline shares findings of its assessment, discusses triggered RAPs, notes resident response to interventions currently in place, shares perspective on problems and needs.

3. Team comes to consensus on problem/need statements for the care plan, measurable goals, specific interventions, and time frames for review of goal status.

Quarterly conference

Held: Following completion of quarterly MDS Assessment.

Attendance: RN responsible for care, social services, activities, and dietary. Others as needed.

- Resident/family/direct care staff may or may not attend dependent on how facility gains involvement of those with resident care.

- Refer to "Care Conference Attendance Involvement" for a detailed discussion of this topic.

Purpose:

- To ensure the interdisciplinary team agrees with the MDS and status of the care plan

- To review care plan effectiveness, modifying and adjusting as needed

RATIONALE	The team must decide if the current goals have been met to evaluate the effectiveness of the plan. Often adjustments to the plan are indicated. If these changes are not made there is a risk of negative outcomes. The team must decide if new needs have occurred. Sometimes a single discipline may be dealing with a problem that other team members are not aware of. Ensuring awareness increases positive outcomes as other disciplines offer varying insights.

Content of the meeting:

1. Overview of the resident course over the past quarter and Quality Indicator results.

2. Review each care plan goal, coming to consensus on status.

3. Each discipline shares findings of its assessment, offers insight, and identifies any additional care planning needs.

4. Discuss status of ADLs, psychoactive drug use, physical restraint use, discharge, and advanced care directives*.

    *These are benchmarks that can directly influence quality of life and quality of care. They are noted here to ensure the facility focuses on review of these items on a regular basis. It is NOT required; rather, it is recommended to provide additional safeguards for the resident and facility.

Significant status change conference

Held: Following completion of the MDS, triggered RAPs review, and professional assessments.

Attendance: RN responsible for care, social services, activities, and dietary. Others as needed.

- Resident/family/direct care staff may or may not attend dependent on how facility gains involvement with resident care.

- Refer to "Care Conference Attendance Involvement" for a detailed discussion of this topic.

Purpose:

- To ensure that the interdisciplinary team is aware of and in agreement with the MDS and RAP decisions

- To review the existing care plan, modifying as needed to reflect the significant changes and plan of action

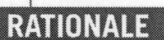 **RATIONALE** When a significant status change occurs, it requires a holistic review of the resident for impact physically, mentally, socially, and emotionally. Each discipline brings a different viewpoint in the assessment process thus ensuring the best results for the resident.

Content of the meeting:

1. Identify the significant change and MDS/RAP findings.

2. Each discipline offers insights and opinion on reason for the change.

3. Discuss alterations to the existing care plan.

© 2009 HCPro, Inc. **The Big Book of Care Plans, Second Edition**

Annual conference

Held: Following completion of the MDS/triggered RAPs, and professional assessments. Annual assessment must be completed within 12 months of the last full MDS/RAP review.

Attendance: RN responsible for care, social services, activities, and dietary.

- Resident/family may or may not attend dependent on how facility gains involvement of all concerned with resident care.

- Please refer to "Care Conference Attendance Involvement" for a detailed discussion related to this topic.

Purpose:

- To ensure the interdisciplinary team agrees with the content of the MDS

- To ensure all team members are in consensus on RAP analysis

- To evaluate the existing care plan; modifying as needed to accommodate findings from yearly review

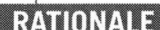 **RATIONALE** Subtle changes occurring over time can accumulate. The yearly assessment and conference ensure the plan stays focused on the resident's actual status.

Content of the meeting:

1. Overview of the course of the resident's care and status over the past year.

2. Discuss the findings of the MDS and RAPs for team consensus.

3. Review the existing plan, status of goals, and appropriateness of interventions.

4. Identify any additional care planning needs.

Room change, re-admission, status check conference

Held: For room changes, re-admissions, and interim reviews prompted by questionable care plan. Interventions when the team is not in agreement about the course of action.

Attendance: RN responsible for care, social services, activities, and dietary.

Purpose:

- To maintain timely assessment and care plan review when conferences are based on room number or other set schedules. If conferences are held based on admission dates and/or last assessment, this conference would not be needed. Read the section on scheduling conferences for more information on this topic.

- To discuss impact of room change on the resident regardless of how conferences are scheduled.

- To review if the care plan put in place is working or requires different approaches.

RATIONALE These conference are a quick review. Staying on target with the care plan is key to maintaining and enhancing status. It is very difficult for one person to hold the accountability for decision-making and ensure a holistic, ongoing appropriate care plan. Room changes often have adverse effects on residents. Re-admissions prompt a need for care plan adjustments even without a significant change. All too often, care plan interventions are not effective. When the team is uncertain of how well a plan will work, a status check is critical.

Content of the meeting:

1. Identify the reason for the review.

2. Designated discipline provides a baseline picture of the resident status.

3. Team validates the existing plan is on target and/or makes the needed adjustments.

Participation and Involvement in Care Planning

Who should participate at scheduled care conferences? When? At what level? Does everybody have to sit down at the same time and place? Federal requirements mandate interdisciplinary care planning.

The intent of the regulation is to ensure that all parties are communicating, and agree to a course of care and plan of action. There are many ways to accomplish this. How you accomplish it is a facility decision. The choice is best made after considering resident and family comfort level, needs, and wants; staffing patterns; time factors; and the pros and cons of the many options available.

You might decide to have several conference levels, with inclusion and exclusions, formal and informal, based on the purpose of the meetings. This does not mean additional time is eaten up—it is more a redistribution of who is involved, when, and at what level.

Resident, family, and direct-care staff attendance at a formal meeting with the professional disciplines is not necessarily the best plan. Residents can feel intimidated and/or uncomfortable talking and being talked about. Often times they will share important information outside of the conference room that has a significant bearing on the care plan. At conference they do not always speak their thoughts, tend to agree when they don't, or go off on tangents unrelated to the discussion. Staff made to attend often have their regular duties interrupted, aren't really sure what their role is, and too frequently are not prepared.

It is imperative to gain resident involvement. Failure to do so renders the plan ineffective. Lack of cooperation in meeting goals, resisting planned interventions, and depersonalization are some of the more important outcomes effected by lack of involvement.

Considerations for involvement in care planning
Participants: Resident, family, and significant other
Assessment:

1. Ask subjective, open-ended questions about the care they receive.

    - Are you satisfied?

    - What would you like to see done differently?

    - Are your needs being met?

    - What do you like best and least about the facility?

    - What changes would you like to see in the plan of care?

 This is an excellent opportunity to educate about the purpose for the care plan.

2. Cognitively impaired residents should also be given the chance to respond. Demented residents often have a theme to their conversation and actions. Can you identify it? Can it be connected with what is going on with them?

3. Call the family prior to conference (whether they are or aren't involved in the meeting). This call needs to be very structured to avoid needless time loss. Always tell them the purpose of the call and how much time it will take. If they get off the subject, redirect. If they bring up problems and concerns unrelated to the purpose of the call, refer them to the appropriate person or tell them you will have that individual call them.

Participants: Floor nurses, nursing assistants, others
Assessment:

1. All shifts need to be included.

2. Dependent on the type of assessment (admission, annual, significant change) some paper tracking is helpful—particularly ADL performance, mood and behavior, bowel and bladder function, intake and output. (**NOTE:** Restorative and rehab programs always require tracking.)

3. Primary caregivers (shift nurse and aide) should be questioned as to resident response to care plan interventions, peculiarities or idiosyncrasies, and general opinion of the resident's status (maintaining, declining, improving), including recommendations.

4. Develop a simple form that all shifts can respond to. This will give the RN assessment nurse a guideline, prompting additional staff input and involvement dependent on the need. Refer to the documentation manual for mood/behavior and ADL tracking tools.

5. These actions should be taken prior to conference, whether these staff members are or are not included in the meeting. This is prep work for care planning. The conference is decision-making time regarding the assessment!

Pros and cons of resident, family, and direct-care staff attendance
Resident/family attendance

1. Provides an opportunity to discuss problems and concerns with the team as a whole. +

2. Can inhibit open, honest discussion of key issues that might be embarrassing or uncomfortable to discuss in a group. −

3. Can bring previously unknown information to the surface. +

4. Eliminates the need for post-conference contact regarding the plan. +

5. Demonstrates facility effort to comply with regulations. +

6. Could foster a positive image of facility concern, care, and services. +

7. Can get off task, missing focus and purpose of the meeting. Families often view it as a time to air their complaints. −

8. Resident often feels intimidated, agrees or contributes little; later shares real thoughts and feelings. −

9. Can absorb significant time if not highly structured and effectively facilitated. −

10. Tends to become more information sharing than problem-solving in focus. −

11. Can create lack of trust and confidence in staff when disagreement or lack of knowledge exists. −

Non-attendance

1. Can result in potential deficiency if other means not initiated to include resident, family in care planning. −

2. Allows professional disagreements to be settled without compromising resident/family confidence. +

3. Encourages free exchange of ideas and opinions on problem causes, goals, and interventions, enabling an on-target, effective care plan to be developed. +

4. Encourages time management and efficiency. +

5. Requires follow-up with resident and family on final plan. −

The questions to be discussed
• Are the positive benefits being realized? If not, why?
• Do the negatives outweigh the positives? Indicating inclusion in care planning by other means.

Care Conference Proceedings

Effective care conferences can only come about with adequate preparation. New admissions take the greatest amount of time. On average, nursing needs two to four hours; other disciplines need one to two hours for assessment and preparation. On a quarterly basis, each resident needs approximately one hour per discipline per quarter. Half of this time is spent in preparation; the remaining time is spent in conference, discussing the resident, finalizing the care plan, and writing the team conference note.

Time management is critical.

The more prepared participants are, the more efficient and effective the conference.

The assessment and care conference lay the foundation for the care plan. The plan is the primary tool for ensuring continuity of care. The care delivered is only as good as the plan developed. It is the professional team's duty to develop and orchestrate the best possible plan, starting with assessment and formalizing at conference. The care plan is the roadmap for primary caregivers. Do your homework!

> ## IF YOU CHOOSE TO INCLUDE FAMILIES IN THE FORMAL CONFERENCE, IT IS RECOMMENDED THAT THE PROFESSIONAL TEAM MEET FIRST WITHOUT THEM.
>
> This allows the team to hammer out disagreements and clarify approaches. The result is a confidence-building presentation for the resident and family and more effective use of time because the team is focused.
>
> The most effective conferences take place when the core participants have specific duties. This enables the care plan to be developed and documented. When conference is over, the documentation is in place. The core team for this purpose consists of the RN Assessment Coordinator, the social worker/designee, the dietitian/diet technician, and the activity therapist/worker.

Before conference

1. Complete the professional assessment: evaluate the resident; talk with caregivers, family, significant others; review the chart.

2. Review the MDS: Do you agree? If not, discuss with RN Assessment Nurse. Are there changes from the previous assessment? What do you see as the problems and needs for care planning?

3. Review the existing plan in its entirety, not just "your stuff." Do you feel problems are accurately stated/addressed? Are goals met? Are they reasonable? Interventions appropriate? Is the plan on target or skirting issues?

4. Create a note card outlining key points you want to address for use as a memory jogger. If something happens and you cannot attend conference, you can have another person share your information, including plans and recommendations.

Remember:

1. If you don't prepare for conference you have wasted valuable time. Knowledge creates empowerment, builds ownership, and enhances credibility. Don't let the resident, the team, or yourself down. Adequate preparation saves many hours over the long run.

2. Review all disciplines' assessments and progress notes, including the physician's. Are you all on the same train? Do you agree? Why or why not? Be ready to discuss these things!

3. If you can't attend conference, regardless of reason, you MUST share your assessment, opinion, and recommendations with another team member. This person can present your information, ensuring your viewpoint is considered.

4. Make preparation a job priority! Block your time. Don't shortchange yourself, the resident, or the team. You are a vital part of successful care planning.

5. If other job duties are preventing you from being an effective care planning participant you will need to review your job duties with your supervisor. After a while, we all collect duties and responsibilities that may not be appropriate.

REVIEW THE DEMANDS OF YOUR JOB.

Calculate the time demands for the care planning process.

If you are responsible for 60 residents, you will need about 20 to 25 hours per month or five to six hours a week to adequately address care planning needs.

Allow one hour per resident per quarter. Determine the average number of admissions each month and give yourself two hours for these.

If you a have a lot of Medicare residents you will need to increase your time allotment as assessments are required more frequently.

Dependent on your facility, the demand on individual disciplines will be different.

During conference

Your goal is to ensure a pertinent, goal-directed care plan. That means everyone participating knows what is expected of them. Adequate knowledge and preparation is accomplished when all the players understand their roles. (Do your grocery list!) Be sure attendees are clear on the purpose, intention, and approximate time commitment.

 This is problem-solving time! Discussion of observations, assessment, analysis, and specific resident needs is the heart of the meeting.

Direct-care staff, if included, must know what is required of them. They will need time to prepare before conference. Conference is NOT the time to leaf through the chart looking for information and mumbling "I don't know". That should be the exception, not the norm!

Finalizing the care plan

Some care plan needs will be in place prior to conference (i.e., admission-risk care plans and plans to address the immediate needs of the resident). At conference these plans may be further modified or even perhaps eliminated. Sometimes clinicians may formulate care plans before conference and bring them to conference. This can save a great deal of time, particularly when the clinician has an excellent working knowledge of the RAP cause-and-effect relationships (for most of us, this is a gradual process). If this path is chosen, individuals, and the team, need to be willing to adapt, modify, scrap, and rewrite the plan if discussion indicates a better or more concise way to address the problems. Please remember that writing plans in advance is never a waste of time. It often gets the ball off the ground at conference!

> **The goal is an easily read and understood, people-friendly care plan that works!**

> **Before you leave conference the plan should be documented and the team progress note written.**

A typical conference including residents and families allows 20 to 30 minutes of talk time and 10 minutes of documentation time. Without resident and family attendance, 20 minutes of talk time and 10 minutes of documentation time is the goal. New admissions can add 10 to 15 minutes to the discussion and refinement of the care plan.

* Medicare PPS conferences are excluded from these time estimates.

Conference roles

Facilitator: Directs, redirects, and keeps the meeting on track. Clarifies, restates care planning decisions for team consensus. Keeps the ball rolling! Professional disciplines can rotate this task if desired.

1. Typically provides overview of the resident, reason for conference, and introduces new faces.

2. Begins requesting attendee input.

   - If resident/family is present, remains sensitive to impact of discussion on them, as well as ensuring terminology is understood. It is a matter of choice and judgment as to when and how to gain their input.

   - Identify MDS findings: triggered RAPs, variances from previous assessment. Have each discipline report its findings AND encourage participants to question, present other viewpoints, etc.

   - Be sure the existing care plan is discussed: problem area, status of goal, need for adjustment, deletion. (It is not necessary that the entire plan be read. A general identification of the problem and the stated goal should provide enough information to prompt discussion and conclusions.)

Timekeeper: Watches the clock! Alerts team of time midway, and when five minutes are remaining. Helps facilitator to redirect team efforts: "There are only five minutes left. Have we addressed the most significant problems?"

Mr./Ms. Clean: Stays out of the "agenda." Identifies attitudes and pitfalls that tend to occur when problems are chronic or difficult to solve. Also restates what has been said so the team can hear what they seem to be saying. Generally the person with the least-vested interest is the most unbiased, and able to hear with fresh ears and new ideas.

Writer: Takes responsibility for writing the team note. Needs to be able to decipher the substance from the trivia. The content of the note reflects reason for meeting, overview of resident status, and rationale for care planning decisions and adjustments to the plan. Reviews the completed note for team; all participants sign agreement.

Plan reviewer: Can be one or several disciplines dependent on how your facility has divided assessment and care planning responsibilities. The reviewer shares content of plan as needed, revises existing plan per team discussion, or combines/rewrites plan per team decision to develop a more interrelated plan. Each discipline can add the interventions for which it will be taking responsibility. The writer's primary responsibility is ensuring that the problem(s) and goal(s) are documented per team decisions. (This task can be combined with any of the above. Mr./Ms. Clean is probably the best combination.)

After conference

All documentation should be in place. It is now time to implement the care plan. This requires COMMUNICATION, EDUCATION, OVERSIGHT, and REVIEW for compliance and effectiveness. The following items must be addressed:

1. Reviewing the plan with the resident and family whenever possible. This can be accomplished via face to face discussions or perhaps phone or letter dependent on facility setup and procedures. If resident and family are disinterested, non-available, etc., record a note to that effect, including what your actions were. If there is no family and/or the resident is incapable of understanding, this can be handled as a one-time-only note, perhaps by social services.

2. Discuss the plan with caregivers across all shifts. Be sure they understand their role and responsibilities and are provided any training they may need.

3. Be sure the team has designated a particular discipline to oversee implementation and effectiveness of the plan. As a rule, the person with the greatest ownership for a problem should oversee the plan. For example, if a resident were significantly depressed, social services or perhaps Activities would oversee plan implementation even though they may not be carrying out the bulk of interventions.

Interdisciplinary Team Progress Report

Resident Name _____ Date _____

Type of Review: Medicare Day: ❏ 5 ❏ 14 ❏ 30 ❏ 60 ❏ 90 ❏ OMRA ❏ Admission ❏ Quarterly ❏ Significant Change ❏ Annual ❏ Other

Quality Indicators that Triggered this Review and Explanation of Relationships/Causes

❏ New Fractures	❏ B&B HR	❏ Fecal Impaction	❏ Dehydration	❏ Psych med HR	❏ Restraints
❏ Falls	❏ B&B LR	❏ UTI	❏ Bedfast	❏ Psych med LR	❏ Little No Activity
❏ HR Behavior	❏ No Toilet-plan	❏ Weight Loss	❏ ADL	❏ Anti-Anxiety	❏ Pressure Ulcer HR
❏ LR Behavior	❏ Catheters	❏ Tube Feeding	❏ ROM	❏ Hypnotic	❏ Pressure Ulcer LR
❏ Depression					
❏ NO RX					
❏ 9+meds					
❏ Cognitive					

If Admit, Significant Change, or Annual Review: Triggered RAPs with Indications for Care Planning

❏ Delirium	❏ ADL/Rehab	❏ Behavior	❏ Nutritional Status	❏ Dental
❏ Cognitive Loss/	❏ Incontinence/Catheter	❏ Restraints	❏ Feeding Tubes	❏ Pressure Ulcer
Dementia	❏ Psychosocial Well Being	❏ Activities	❏ Dehydration/Fluid	❏ Psychotropic Drug Use
❏ Vision	❏ Mood	❏ Falls	Maintenance	
❏ Communication				

Immediate Need Care Plan Patterns/Trends If Applicable This Review

Interdisciplinary Team Progress Report (cont.)

Directions: Begin by summarizing the resident's status inclusive of Quality Indicators Triggered and clinical relationships of the indicators to each other, if present. If an admission, significant change, or annual review, note the causal relationships of RAPs to each other with indications for care planning.

Include: Summary of Status,   QI Clinical Relationships,   RAP Clinical Relationships

_____
_____
_____
_____
_____
_____
_____
_____
_____
_____
_____
_____
_____
_____
_____
_____
_____
_____
_____
_____
_____
_____
_____
_____
_____
_____
_____
_____
_____
_____

       The Big Book of Care Plans, Second Edition

Interdisciplinary Team Progress Report (cont.)

STATUS OF CORE CARE PLAN GOALS AND MODIFICATIONS/ADDITIONS

Goal codes: **A** = Goal met, discontinue plan   **B** = Goal Met, continue plan for maintenance   **C** = Goal not met, plan revised/adjusted

Problem/Need Area or Plan Number	Goal Status	Rationale for Actions/Plan Changes/Additions (if other than goal met, discontinue plan)

Interdisciplinary Team Progress Report (cont.)

CARE PLAN, CONFERENCE, AND DISCUSSION ATTENDED BY AND/OR INCLUDED:

Facility Personnel Signature	Discipline	❏ Resident ❏ Family ❏ Next of kin ❏ Significant other
		❏ Provided input prior to conference
		❏ Unable to attend, report mailed post-conference
		❏ Reviewed verbally post-conference with
		_____
		❏ Resident unable ❏ No interested parties
		❏ Attended, Signature below

Federal Regulatory Requirement

Refer to F-Tag #272 §483.20: <u>Resident Assessment.</u>

To provide the facility with ongoing assessment information necessary to develop a care plan, to provide the appropriate care and services for each resident, and to modify the care plan and care/services based on the resident's status.

The facility is expected to use resident observation and communication as the primary source of information when completing the RAI. In addition to direct observation and communication with the resident, the facility should use a variety of other sources, including communication with licensed and non-licensed staff members on all shifts and may include discussions with the resident's physician, family members, or outside consultants and review of the resident's record.

F-Tag #271 (a) <u>Admission Orders.</u>

At the time each resident is admitted, the facility must have physician orders for the resident's immediate care.

§483.20(a) <u>Guidelines:</u>

"Physician orders for immediate care" are those written orders facility staff need to provide essential care to the resident, consistent with the resident's mental and physical status upon admission. These orders should, at a minimum, include dietary, drugs (if necessary), and routine care to maintain or improve the resident's functional abilities until staff can conduct a comprehensive assessment and develop an interdisciplinary care plan.

F-Tag #272 (b) Comprehensive Assessments.

(1) Resident Assessment Instrument. A facility must make a comprehensive assessment of a resident's needs, using the RAI specified by the State. The assessment must include at least the following:

§483.20(b) Intent:

To ensure that the RAI is used in conducting comprehensive assessments as part of an ongoing process through which the facility identifies the resident's functional capacity and health status.

§483.20(b) Guidelines:

The facility is responsible for addressing all needs and strengths of residents regardless of whether the issue is included in the MDS or RAPs. The scope of the RAI does not limit the facility's responsibility to assess and address all care needed by the resident.

Furthermore, the facility is responsible for addressing the resident's needs from the moment of admission.

"Documentation of summary information (xvii) regarding the additional assessment performed through the resident assessment protocols (RAPs)" corresponds to MDS v. 2.0 Section V, and refers to documentation concerning which RAPs have been triggered, documentation of assessment information in support of clinical decision-making relevant to the RAP, documentation regarding where, in the clinical record, information related to the RAP can be found, and for each triggered RAP, whether the identified problem was included in the care plan.

(xviii) Documentation of participation in assessment.

"Documentation of participation in the assessment" corresponds to MDS v. 2.0 Section R, and refers to documentation of who participated in the assessment process. The assessment process must include direct observation and communication with the resident, as well as communication with licensed and non-licensed direct care staff members on all shifts.

F273 (2) *when required*. A facility must conduct a comprehensive assessment of a resident as follows:

(i) Within 14 calendar days after admission, excluding readmissions in which there is no significant change in the resident's physical or mental condition. (For purposes of this section, "readmission" means a return to the facility following a temporary absence for hospitalization or for therapeutic leave.)

§483.20(b)(2) Intent:

To assess residents in a timely manner.

F274 (ii) Within 14 days after the facility determines, or should have determined, that there has been a significant change in the resident's physical or mental condition. (For purpose of this section, a "significant change" means a major decline or improvement in the resident's status that will not normally resolve itself without further intervention by staff or by implementing standard disease-related clinical interventions, that has an impact on more than one area of the resident's health status, and requires interdisciplinary review or revision of the care plan, or both.)

§483.20(b)(2)(ii) Guidelines:

The following are the criteria for significant changes:
A significant change reassessment is generally indicated if decline or improvement is consistently noted in two or more areas of decline or two or more areas of improvement:

Decline:

- Any decline in activities of daily living (ADL) physical functioning where a resident is newly coded as 3, 4 or 8 Extensive assistance, Total dependency, Activity did not occur (note that even if coding in both columns A and B of an ADL category changes, this is considered one ADL change);

- Increase in the number of areas where Behavioral Symptoms are coded as "not easily altered" (e.g., an increase in the use of code 1's for E4B);

- Resident's decision-making changes from 0 or 1, to 2 or 3;

- Resident's incontinence pattern changes from 0 or 1 to 2, 3, or 4, or placement of an indwelling catheter;

- Emergence of sad or anxious mood as a problem that is not easily altered;

- Emergence of an unplanned weight loss problem (5% change in 30 days or 10% change in 180 days);

- Begin to use trunk restraint or a chair that prevents rising for a resident when it was not used before;

- Emergence of a condition/disease in which a resident is judged to be unstable;

- Emergence of a pressure ulcer at Stage II or higher, when no ulcers were previously present at Stage II or higher; or

- Overall deterioration of resident's condition; resident receives more support (e.g., in ADLs or decision-making).

Improvement:

- Any improvement in ADL physical functioning where a resident is newly coded as 0, 1, or 2 when previously scored as a 3, 4, or 8;

- Decrease in the number of areas where Behavioral Symptoms or Sad or Anxious Mood are coded as "not easily altered;"

- Resident's decision making changes from 2 or 3, to 0 or 1;

- Resident's incontinence pattern changes from 2, 3, or 4 to 0 or 1; or

- Overall improvement of resident's condition; resident receives fewer supports.

If the resident experiences a significant change in status, the next annual assessment is not due until 366 days after the significant change reassessment has been completed.

F-Tag #278 (g) Accuracy of Assessment. The assessment must accurately reflect the resident's status.

(h) Coordination. A registered nurse must conduct or coordinate each assessment with the appropriate participation of health professionals.

(i) Certification.

(1) A registered nurse must sign and certify that the assessment is completed.

(2) Each individual who completes a portion of the assessment must sign and certify the accuracy of that portion of the assessment.

(j) Penalty for falsification.
    (1) Under Medicare and Medicaid, an individual who willfully and knowingly—
        (i) Certifies a material and false statement in a resident assessment is subject to a civil money penalty of not more than $1,000 for each assessment; or
        (ii) Causes another individual to certify a material and false statement in a resident assessment is subject to a civil money penalty or not more than $5,000 for each assessment.

    (2) Clinical disagreement does not constitute a material and false statement.

§483.20(g) Intent:

To assure that each resident receives an accurate assessment by staff that are qualified to assess relevant care areas and knowledgeable about the resident's status and needs.

§483.20(g) Guidelines:

"The accuracy of the assessment" means that the appropriate, qualified health professional correctly documents the resident's medical, functional, and psychosocial problems and identifies resident strengths to maintain or improve medical status, functional abilities, and psychosocial status.

The initial comprehensive assessment provides baseline data for ongoing assessment of resident progress.

§483.20(h) Intent:

The registered nurse will conduct and/or coordinate the assessment, as appropriate. Whether conducted or coordinated by the registered nurse, he or she is responsible for certifying that the assessment has been completed.

<u>§483.20(h) Guidelines:</u>

According to the Utilization Guidelines for each state's RAI, the physical, mental, and psychosocial condition of the resident determines the appropriate level of involvement of physicians, nurses, rehabilitation therapists, activities professionals, medical social workers, dietitians, and other professionals, such as developmental disabilities specialists, in assessing the resident. Involvement of other disciplines is dependent upon resident status and needs.

<u>§483.20(g)(h) Probes:</u>

- Have appropriate health professionals assessed the resident? For example, has the resident's nutritional status been assessed by someone who is knowledgeable in nutrition and capable of correctly assessing a resident?

- If the resident's medical status, functional abilities, or psychosocial status declined and the decline was not clinically unavoidable, were the appropriate health professionals involved in assessing the resident?

- Based on your total review of the resident, is each portion of the assessment accurate?

MDS Supporting Documentation

Introduction

Increasing regulatory scrutiny, high demand for quality documentation that supports the MDS 2.0 coding, and the need to clearly reflect clinically unavoidable problems in the medical record is essential. The forms and formats in this manual have been designed to support MDS coding and validate clinical decision-making. When used as designed you will find these tools not only enhance resident outcomes but also meet the test of regulatory scrutiny.

Comprehensive Professional Assessments in this manual will support MDS coding and provide clear rationale for decision-making when completed in their entirety. These assessments will eliminate doubling back to complete RAPs triggered by the MDS because the related RAP guidelines have been incorporated into the assessments. Eleven of the 18 RAPs are covered in the professional assessments for nursing, social services, dietary, and activities. Quarterly assessments for dietary, social services, and activities are standardized and designed to support MDS coding and ensure critical information is collected.

Tracking tools for the direct-care staff and unit nurses are laid out in a user-friendly format. Their use will further enhance accurate MDS coding and aid in communication among and between disciplines. Trackers allow social services, dietary, and activities to complete their assessments in a more flexible time frame as the trackers ensure data is collected through the assessment reference date. Any variance in information on the trackers from the professional assessments can alert the disciplines to resident changes, differences in perception, or perhaps the resident's performance or behavior shifts depending on who was doing the assessment. In any case, the trackers will always facilitate communication.

The structured, user-oriented care plan format provides clear direction for its users. It is designed to flow with the MDS and flag changes when used in the suggested care plan format. Individual RAP guidelines for each of the 18 RAPs are presented in a format designed to facilitate clinically appropriate decision-making. The forms are structured to encourage analysis of collected data and use standardized prompts to encourage completion of critical elements surveyors and outside reviewers look for.

Every effort has been made to ensure information is accurate and as up to date as possible. The user is cautioned to keep abreast of ongoing changes and clarifications and assumes full responsibility for use of the information and documentation tools in this manual. Regardless of what type of documentation format is used, it still takes the individual reviewer's expertise to complete and then analyze the information. Forms that are well constructed can go a long way toward assisting in an effective review.

Recommendations and Rationale for Use of Forms

New admissions and annual reviews

All disciplines: Nursing, dietary, social services, and activities

I.   Complete full assessments which contain designated RAP guidelines. If any of the designated RAPs trigger following completion of the MDS, it will NOT be necessary to complete additional assessment tools or paper work.

Nursing admission/annual assessment contains RAP guidelines for vision, communication, and dental: The admitting nurse may collect the information. An RN should review the admission assessment for completion, making any additional analysis and decision-making as needed. The RN can add additional documentation to the form along with date and signature.

Social service assessment contains RAP guidelines for cognition, mood behavior, and well being: It is important that ALL information be recorded. Do NOT skip sections. If information is unknown or not available, indicate this on the form. Once you have collected all the data, review the information and note your rationale for proceeding or not proceeding to care planning in the designated section. Review the completed MDS to ensure you are in consensus. This must be done prior to the MDS being locked and preferably prior to care conference.

On occasion, tracking information completed by the nursing department may not be in concert with your assessment. You will need to determine if the resident is now different from when you completed your assessment. If this is the case, make a brief progress note indicating your awareness and indicate if any changes need to be made to your initial care planning decisions.

Dietary assessment contains RAP guidelines for nutrition, hydration, and tube feeding:

It is important that ALL information be recorded. Do NOT skip sections. If information is unknown or not available, indicate this on the form. Once you have collected all the data, review the information and note your rationale for proceeding or not proceeding to care planning in the designated section. Review the completed MDS to ensure you are in consensus. This must be done prior to the MDS being locked and preferably prior to care conference.

On occasion, tracking information completed by the nursing department may not be in concert with your assessment. You will need to determine if the resident is now different from when you completed your assessment. If this is the case, make a brief progress note indicating your awareness and indicate if any changes need to be made to your initial care planning decisions.

Activities assessment contains activity RAP:

It is important that ALL information be recorded. Do NOT skip sections. If information is unknown or not available, indicate this on the form. Once you have collected all the data, review the information and note your rationale for proceeding or not proceeding to care planning in the designated section.

Review the completed MDS to ensure you are in consensus. This must be done prior to the MDS being locked and preferably prior to care conference. On occasion, tracking information completed by the nursing department may not be in concert with your assessment. You will need to determine if the resident is now different from when you completed your assessment. If this is the case, make a brief progress note indicating your awareness and indicate if any changes need to be made to your initial care planning decisions.

II. On the RAP summary sheet, simply note location of information on the triggered RAP as the professional assessment, including the date of that assessment.

III. Designated person completes the individual "standalone" RAPs. The rationale is noted below. Place the RAP analysis sheet on the back of each individual RAP Evaluation.

ADL RAP. This RAP will always be triggered unless the resident is independent in all areas. Consequently it is not necessary to wait until the MDS has been completed to do this RAP.

Remember, one individual may collect the data and another individual may analyze the information. If this is the case, be sure each person signs and dates the portion he or she has completed.

On the RAP summary sheet note location of information as "ADL RAP dated ____."

Skin RAP and Fall RAP are best completed on the first day of admission. Although they may not trigger on the MDS, these are high-risk areas and always a point of emphasis during survey. The forms are set up to provide a numerical rating that will prompt initiation of a care plan if at-risk score is present. Instruct the user to circle all applicable items that determined the score. Be sure a written analysis is completed as well (place the form on the back of the RAP). Though not mandated per se, it will ensure the facility has reviewed all pertinent factors and minimize questioning by outside reviewers. Even if these RAPs do not trigger on the MDS you will want to note on the RAP summary sheet if you have proceeded. CMS has asked that you do this. Make a brief note that it did not trigger on the MDS to avoid confusion for others who may be correlating the summary sheet with the triggered RAP.

Remember, one individual may collect the data and another individual may analyze the information. If this is the case, be sure each person signs and dates the portion he or she has completed.

On the RAP summary sheet note location of information as "Fall RAP dated ____" and "Skin RAP dated ____."

Physical Restraint RAP. CMS regulations demand an assessment prior to using a physical restraint; the law further demands that medical need be established. Therefore, if you have an order for restraints or are considering their use, complete the Restraint RAP. If you use a restraint, the MDS will trigger the RAP. This will eliminate a double-back step. The format in the manual ensures all essential elements of the review are covered when completed as designed.

On the RAP summary sheet note location of information as "Physical Restraint RAP dated ____."

Psychoactive Drug RAP. If psychoactive meds are in use the RAP will always trigger. If admitted on a psychoactive medication initiating this RAP early in the admission process can help establish a baseline and aid in determining continuing need and possibly medication side effects. The analysis of this RAP is structured to ensure you meet regulatory guidelines on the use of these meds.

On the RAP summary sheet note location of information as "Psychoactive Drug RAP dated ____."

Urinary Incontinence/Catheters RAP. Complete this anytime in the 14-day assessment process. If incontinence or a catheter is present, you already know it will trigger on the MDS. Therefore, the sooner you can evaluate, the sooner you can assure the better outcomes.

On the RAP summary sheet note location of information as "Urinary Incontinence RAP or Catheter RAP dated ____."

Delirium RAP. This is a broad screening RAP. That means it triggers very easily. It is important to carefully review each of the guidelines to determine if there are definite causes or contributing factors that account for the resident's mental changes and variances. It is recommended that nursing complete this RAP, as medical causes are the first rule-out to be done.

On the RAP summary sheet note location of information as "Delirium RAP dated ____."

Quarterly reviews and significant change reviews

Nursing

Nursing does not need to do a specific assessment for MDS quarterly reviews or significant changes. Nursing is conducting assessments on an ongoing basis via nurse's notes and care plan entries.

Use of the <u>ADL and Mood and Behavior Trackers</u> will ensure up-to-the-minute snapshot status for the MDS assessment reference date (ARD). These trackers should be initiated six days prior to the ARD and completed through the ARD.

The <u>Comprehensive Nurses' Summary</u>, though not mandated, is an excellent way to keep the direct-care nurse and assistant involved with the process. It is suggested that these be completed once each month on a rotating-shift basis using the ADL Directive as the comparative tool for decisions on resident current status. If there are variances, they should be reported to the MDS Coordinator who can then determine if a significant status change may be present.

The <u>Immediate Needs Care Plan</u> addresses those problems and needs that may come and go during the quarter as well as unstable conditions that require regular monitoring. Nurse's notes at some frequency will always accompany these plans. A review of these in conjunction with the MDS being completed will further ensure accuracy and identification of any developing trends that may require action.

If a significant change is present, once the MDS is completed and RAPs triggered (or you know a particular RAP will trigger), complete individual RAPs based on assigned discipline.

Social services, dietary, activities

Complete the quarterly/periodic assessment form for your discipline. These quarterly assessments are designed to support the MDS coding. They can be done in the time frame decided by your facility prior to the MDS ARD.

As long as the ADL and Mood Behavior trackers are being used in the MDS ARD window it is not necessary for every discipline to use the same date on their assessment, thereby allowing a more comprehensive evaluation for the quarter. If there are conflicts with the trackers there must be communication, and it may require an additional short note by the affected discipline to ensure everyone is in concert. These conflicts can be easily resolved if each discipline reviews the MDS prior to locking. And, of course, the MDS Coordinator is the double assurance validator alerting others to possible conflicts as he or she correlates information.

If a significant status change is present, you can use this assessment and then complete any triggered RAPs assigned to you by using the individual RAP format located in this manual.

RAP Evaluation for Activities of Daily Living

Name _____ **Date** _____

Directions: For EACH ITEM indicate if it is a Strength or Problem, or if it presents or not. Add any clarifying information in the comments section. Review completed information, considering the relationship of problems, strengths, and other problems present to determine care planning decisions.

REHAB / RESTORABILITY	PROBLEM	STRENGTH	CLARIFYING INFORMATION
Able to make decisions in depth			
Able to make decisions with difficulty			
Decision-making poor, requires supervision, cues			
Rarely/never makes decisions			
Able to understand all/most of time			
Vision adequate to perform (with or without glasses)			
Coordination/dexterity intact			
Able to balance sitting and standing			
Has the ability to learn/remember			
Has the ability to follow directions			
CONDITION / OTHER FACTORS	**YES**	**NO**	**CLARIFYING INFORMATION**
Acute confusion (Delirium)			See related RAP
Symptoms of Depression (MDS Section E)			If YES, how does it impact on ADL performance?
Behavior problems not easily altered ❑ Verbally/physically abusive ❑ Care resistance			If YES, what are they and how do they impact ADLs?
Health status unstable			If YES, does it prevent restorative care?
Status varies over course of day			If YES, why and what is the window of opportunity?
Motivated to work at restorative program			
Mood-altering drugs in use (Psychoactive meds)			If YES, what is effect on ADL?
Medical conditions contributing to need for ADL support ❑ CVA ____ Hemi ____ Para ❑ Parkinson's ❑ CHF ❑ COPD Other _____			

Expected course is to ❑ Improve status ❑ Maintain status ❑ Slow decline
❑ Prevent complications of _____
Refer to ❑ OT ❑ PT ❑ Speech/Language ❑ Restorative nursing ❑ Direct-care staff

Signature/Title of evaluator or person completing RAP _____

RAP Evaluation for Cognitive Loss/Dementia

Name _____ Date _____

Directions: For EACH ITEM, indicate if it is present or not. Add any clarifying information, then review all information, considering if check indicates a problem or strength and the relationship to and need for care planning. Using the data to validate your decision to proceed or not, document your analysis on the reverse side of this document.

	YES	NO	CLARIFYING INFORMATION
Presence of neurological disease Alzheimer's			
Other dementias			
Delirium			
MR/DD			
Factors that can worsen, interact with, or suggest reversible causes Concurrent medical problems			
CVA			
CHF			
COPD, emphysema, asthma			
Cancer			
Diabetes			
Hyperthyroidism			
Medications Started, stopped, changed last 30 days			
Use of antipsychotics (Indicate reason for use)			
Use of hypnotics (Indicate if "hangover" effect)			
Use of antidepressants (Indicate length of time receiving)			
Mood/behavior factors Sadness, withdrawn from activities, signs of mood distress			
Dx of depression/manic depression (Indicate if symptomatic)			
Anxiety or other psychiatric disorder			
Inappropriate actions/behavior			
Resist care; difficulty/inability to comprehend what is asked or done			
Unable to distinguish what is or isn't theirs; takes things from others			
Wanders in and out of other rooms			
Becomes verbally/physically abusive when asked/directed to do something			
Additional considerations for care planning Physical restraints used			
Hearing/vision deficit			
Ability to understand compromised			
ADL compromised			
B&B function compromised			
Terminal prognosis/failure to thrive			

Signature/Title of evaluator or person completing RAP _____

RAP Evaluation for Psychosocial Well Being

Name _____ Date _____

Directions: For EACH ITEM, indicate if it is present or not. Add any clarifying information, then review all information, considering if check indicates a problem or strength and the relationship to and need for care planning. Using the data to validate your decision to proceed or not, document your analysis on the reverse side of this document.

	YES	NO	N/A	CLARIFYING INFORMATION
Were mood or behavior problems present before reduced sense of well being?				
Do mood or behavior problems impact on sense of well being?				
Have previous or current interventions or treatment programs been effective?				

	YES	NO	CLARIFYING INFORMATION
Have key social relationships been terminated or altered (e.g. loss of family, friends, or others)?			
Have external factors impacted on well being (e.g., use of restraints change in room/mate, recent admission)?			
Do cognitive or communication deficits or lack of interest in activities impede interaction with others?			
Is resident uncomfortable in social/group settings?			
Was life more satisfactory prior to admission)?			
Is there preoccupation with past or unwillingness to acknowledge the present?			
Does staff or resident perceive this to be a serious problem?			
Are corrective strategies now in use?			
Is this an area that might be improved?			

Signature/Title of evaluator or person completing RAP _____

RAP Evaluation for Mood

Name _____ Date _____

Directions: For EACH ITEM, indicate if it is present or not. Add any clarifying information, then review all information, considering if check indicates a problem or strength and the relationship to and need for care planning. Using the data to validate your decision to proceed or not, document your analysis on the reverse side of this document.

	YES	NO	CLARIFYING INFORMATION
New/worsening conditions that may be affecting mood			
Alzheimer's disease			
Cancer			
Metabolic/endocrine disorders (e.g., Parkinson's, neurological disease, thyroid disease, hypoglycemis, hypokalemia, stroke, Cushings, Addison's disease)			
Dx manic depression or anxiety disorder or other psychiatric disorder or cycles of decline/improvement			
Potentially reversible causes that may be affecting mood			
Sudden onset or worsening of cognitive or communication problems since starting new meds or treatments			
Taking medications known to cause mood shifts (e.g., psychotropic, sedatives, stimulants, cataprees, ismelin, aldomet, inderal, tagamet, cytotoxic agents, digitalis, immuno suppressants, steroids)			
Other potential complicating factors			
Acute confusion (delirium)			
Recent change in life, death of loved one or changes in environment, or catastrophic illness, etc.			
Problems with relationships			
Poor sleep quality/quantity			
ADL decline PRIOR to mood problem			
ADL decline AFTER mood problem			
Communication difficulties affect mood			
Initiative/response to interventions			
Takes little or no initiative			
Sad mood is persistent			
Mood relatively unchanged last 90 days			
Receiving medication for mood			
Receiving counseling for mood			
Mood improved with current treatment			

Signature/Title of Evaluator or person completing RAP _____

RAP Evaluation for Behavior

Name _____ Date _____

Directions: For EACH ITEM, indicate if it is present or not. Add any clarifying information, then review all information, considering if check indicates a problem or strength and the relationship to and need for care planning. Using the data to validate your decision to proceed or not, document your analysis on the reverse side of this document.

	YES	NO	CLARIFYING INFORMATION
Potential factors affecting behavior			
Acute health condition			
Reaction to medication (started, stopped, changed last 30–90 days)			
Neurological disorder			
Cognitive impairment with comprehension difficulties			
Declining cognitive status			
Mood problems			
Relationship problems			
Physical restraints used			
Psychoactive drugs used			
Environmental stressors (e.g., too loud, noisy, or too quiet)			
Sensory impairments: hearing, vision, touch, etc.			
Psychiatric condition			
Transfer to new unit			
Change in room/mate			
Change in personnel			
Does behavior problem occur with care interventions?			
Does behavior create difficulty with people? If yes, in what way?			
Does behavior interfere with self-performance or treatment regimens?			
Does behavior endanger or distress the resident or others? If yes, how?			
Behavior is verbally abusive. If yes, indicate circumstances.			
Behavior is physically aggressive. If yes, indicate circumstances.			
Behavior is socially inappropriate. If yes, indicate how.			
Behavior is wandering. If yes, explain why this is a problem.			
Is there a pattern to the behavior? (certain time, place, people, circumstances precipitate the problem)			

Signature/Title of evaluator or person completing RAP _____

Psychotropic Drug RAP Assessment

Name _____ Date _____

I. HISTORY

Classes of drugs in use ❑ Antipsychotic ❑ Anti-anxiety ❑ Antidepressants ❑ Hypnotics

Drug name	Frequency	Reason prescribed	Length of time remaining

Problems with metabolism/excretion ❑ Acute condition ❑ Dehydration/fluid intake ❑ Impaired liver/kidney function

Current status mood/behavior ❑ Stable ❑ Declining ❑ Improving ❑ Resolved

Psychiatric condition(s) present ❑ No ❑ Yes, _____

Non-medical management plan in place ❑ No ❑ Yes Comments _____

II. GUIDELINES TO CONSIDER Mark yes or no. Use comments section to clarify.

Guideline	Yes	No	Comments
Depression present or worsened			
Decline in mood/behavior ADL			
Hallucinations/delusions present or worsened			
Cognition worse or recently impaired			
Acute confusion not r/t to severe depression/medical illness			
Sedation or drowsiness since med(s)			
Slurred speech			
Gait/balance disturbance			
Urinary incontinence worsened or recently developed			
Falls			
Dry mouth			
General status decline since med(s)			
Risk factors explained, understood, and agreed to by resident/family/guardian			

III. POTENTIAL ANTIPSYCHOTIC DRUG-RELATED SIDE EFFECTS

Only do this if on antipsych. med. If YES to any, complete standardized test for involuntary movements such as AIMS.

Orthostatic hypotension Systolic drop 20 pts sit to stand or c/o dizziness, loss of balance from lying to sit/stand position			
Tremors, unsteadiness, pill rolling. Rigidity of limb, neck, trunk, or shuffling gait			
Akinesia: marked decrease in spontaneous movement			
Dystonia: holds self in rigid unnatural position			
Akathisia: unable to sit still			
Tardive dyskenesia: involuntary movements (e.g., thrusting, chewing movements)			
Parkinson's disease			

Signature/Title of evaluator or person completing RAP _____

 The Big Book of Care Plans, Second Edition

Analysis, Decision-Making, and Consent Regarding Psychoactive Medication

Antipsychotics

If condition is not controlled or improved without significant drug side effect, a dose adjustment or different medication may be indicated. If none of the below conditions is present, use of this drug category is generally contraindicated.

❑ Major mental illness or disorder.
❑ Psychotic symptoms, causing frightful distress (hallucinations, delusions, paranoia resulting in significant dysfunction).
❑ Organic mental syndrome, exhibiting behaviors harmful to self or interfering with staff ability to perform necessary care.

Antidepressants

❑ Symptoms of depression are present.　　　　　　　　　　　　**Geriatric depression scale score:** _____
❑ Medication is new and/or given less than 30 days; time is needed to determine effectiveness.
❑ Continues to exhibit signs of depression, medication adjustment to be discussed with physician.
❑ Symptoms of depression are not present.　　　　　　　　　**Geriatric depression scale score:** _____
❑ Medication has been/is effective in controlling symptoms of depression.
❑ No previous history of depression prior to this, physician will evaluate continuing need every _____ months.
❑ History of recurrent depression, continued use is appropriate in absence of significant side effects.

Anti-Anxiety (If none of the below conditions is present, use of this drug category is generally contraindicated.)

❑ Neuromuscular syndromes (cerebral palsy, tardive dyskinesia, seizure disorder)
❑ General anxiety disorder
❑ Organic mental syndrome creating distress/dysfunction or danger to self or others
❑ Symptomatic anxiety occurring with other diagnosed psychiatric disorder (depression, adjustment disorder, etc.)
❑ Other _____

Hypnotic/Sedatives (Continued use more than 10 days is contraindicated.)

❑ Poor sleep habits　　❑ Given to establish sleep　　❑ Resident request/demands　　❑ Other _____

ANALYSIS FOR CARE PLANNING

DOSE ADJUSTMENT　❑ Indicated/underway
❑ Not anticipated lowest dose possible to manage symptoms, continued care planning for risk monitoring.
IF DRUG SIDE EFFECTS ARE PRESENT PHYSICIAN ACTION TAKEN/REQUESTED. (If not, why not and plan)
❑ NA　　❑ Lower dose　　❑ Different medication　　❑ Additional med added to control side effects

Summarize the impact of medication use on functional status. Identify the specific behaviors or symptoms being treated or managed with the medication(s). Indicate what actions will be taken, any complications, risk, or referrals that may be indicated. Use the information on the reverse side to assist in determining the best course of action. If resident/family is not in agreement, note reasons and plan.

_____
_____
_____

CONSENT: ❑ Yes　　❑ No　　　　BY: ❑ Resident　　❑ Family　　❑ Guardian
Agree to use and plan developed. Parties sign below.

_____ **Date** _____
_____ **Date** _____

Signature/Title of evaluator or person completing RAP _____

RAP Evaluation for Delirium

Name _____ Date _____

Directions: For EACH ITEM, indicate if it is present or not. Add any clarifying information, then review all information, considering if check indicates a problem or strength and the relationship to and need for care planning. Using the data to validate your decision to proceed or not, document your analysis on the reverse side of this document.

	YES	NO	CLARIFYING INFORMATION
Changes from baseline status Difficulty breathing			
BP +/- 20 points from baseline or BP less than 100 with usual BP more than 100			
Pulse rate +/- 20 points from baseline or < 50 / > 130			
Fecal impaction is present			
Urine output < 400 cc / 24 hrs, or 150 cc / shift or less			
Blood sugar < 50 – 70 If so, check for liver abnormality and diabetes			
Change in lab values from baseline			
Recent head injury or fall			
Food intake < 50% from baseline x 3 days			
Sleep problems/disturbances			
Medication considerations Any meds started, stopped, or changed in last 30 days			
Potential drug interactions. Review drug profile with pharmacist			
Taking more than one drug from same class (e.g. psychotropics)			
Psychosocial considerations Isolated from others, objects, situations (e.g., recent hospitalization, living alone, loss of valued object)			
Confused about time, place, people			
Recent loss of family, friend, care taker, loved one			
Recent increase in sadness, depression, anxious mood			
Physical restraint used			
Recent change in environment (e.g., room/mate, new to NF, was in hospital, etc.)			
Sensory losses Hearing deficits, wax impacted in ears, or hearing aid dysfunction			
Vision deficits without correction			
Sensory deprivation: little or no stimulation			
Environment lacks personalization with familiar items			
Dx Alzheimer's/dementia with rapid worsening			

Signature/Title of evaluator or person completing RAP _____

RAP Evaluation for Visual Function

Name _____ Date _____

Directions: For EACH ITEM, indicate if it is present or not. Add any clarifying information, then review all information, considering if check indicates a problem or strength and the relationship to and need for care planning. Using the data to validate your decision to proceed or not, document your analysis on the reverse side of this document.

	YES	NO	CLARIFYING INFORMATION
Diagnosis/medication			
Diabetes			
Cataracts			
Glaucoma/macular degeneration			
Eye medication, received as ordered			NA
Has side effects from eye medication			NA
Complains of eye pain, blurred vision, double vision, or sudden loss of vision			
Eye exam since problem noted			
Seen by ophthalmologist/optometrist. If no, why (e.g., unable to cooperate, refused, etc.)?			
If neurological problem or dementia, exam done for visual/perceptual problems			
Recommendations made and followed			NA
Functional need for eye exam or new glasses			
Vision problem interferes with ability to eat, walk unassisted, interact with others			
Vision limits ability to recognize others			
Difficulty negotiating environment or participating in self-care activities			
Difficulty seeing TV or reading			
Expresses interest in improved vision			
Environmental factors/care planning considerations			
Complains of visual difficulties since being in new environment			
Environment adapted to need (e.g., large print signs, phone numbers, 300-watt reading lamp)			
Could be more independent with visual cues (e.g., labeling, task segmentation, sensory cues such as cane to recognize objects in pathway, etc.)			
Glasses labeled or color coded in a way that resident/staff know when they are to be used			
Lenses clean/free of scratches			
Glasses were used and are now lost			

Signature/Title of evaluator or person completing RAP _____

RAP Evaluation for Communication

Name _____ Date _____

Directions: For EACH ITEM, indicate if it is present or not. Add any clarifying information, then review all information, considering if check indicates a problem or strength and the relationship to and need for care planning. Using the data to validate your decision to proceed or not, document your analysis on the reverse side of this document.

	YES	NO	CLARIFYING INFORMATION
Communication components to consider Visual function impaired and not compensated (e.g., glasses, environment, etc.)			
Recent change in hearing or impaired hearing			
Impacted ear wax			
Ear drainage			
Hearing is adequate for conversational tone			
Evaluated by audiologist if hearing is impaired			NA
Condition worsened since last visit			NA
Recommendations made and followed. If no, indicate why.			NA
Has and uses hearing aid. If not indicate why.			
Resident/staff familiar with use (i.e., battery checks, volume control, etc.)			
Speech is clear			
Able to understand			
Able to be understood			
Are opportunities available to communicate? Are there people to talk to?			
Problems requiring further assessment or resolution if present			
Decline in cognitive status			
Decline in ADL status			
Decline in mood or increasing problems with mood			

Signature/Title of evaluator or person completing RAP _____

RAP Evaluation for Dental Care

Name _____ Date _____

Directions: For EACH ITEM, indicate if it is present or not. Add any clarifying information, then review all information, considering if check indicates a problem or strength and the relationship to and need for care planning. Using the data to validate your decision to proceed or not, document your analysis on the reverse side of this document.

	YES	NO	CLARIFYING INFORMATION
Problem factors to consider			
Mouth pain or sensitivity is present			
Lesions, ulcers, inflammation, bleeding, swelling, or rashes present			
Pain, fever, or swollen glands present			
Candidiasis; white areas in mouth			
Teeth broken, loose, missing, or carious			
Denture pain or complaints about dentures			NA
Does not have or will not wear dentures/partials			NA
Complains about the taste of many foods. If yes, indicate if medication cause has been ruled out.			
Leaves 25% or more of food uneaten. If yes, indicate if oral/dental problems have been ruled out as causative factors.			
Lips, tongue, or mouth are dry, sticky, or coated with film			
Taking meds that cause dry mouth (e.g., decongestants, antihistamines, diuretics, antihypertensives, antidepressants, antipsychotics, etc.)			
If dry mouth, have these interventions been tried: saliva substitute, lip balm, increasing fluid intake?			
Self image could benefit from dental interventions			
Resist mouth care related to lack of motivation, depression, pain, staff approach, never caring for teeth/mouth in past			
Functional considerations			
Needs reminders to brush teeth			
Can follow verbal directions/demonstrations for mouth care			
Need task segmentation to perform			
Vision adequate to perform oral care			
Hand dexterity adequate to perform oral care			
Motivated to perform oral care			
Medical problems of dental concern			
Rheumatic Fever, Valvular Heart Disease, Anticoagulant use, Hip Replacement, Diabetes			

Signature/Title of evaluator or person completing RAP _____

The Big Book of Care Plans, Second Edition   © 2009 HCPro, Inc.

RAP Evaluation for Nutrition

Name _____ Date _____

Directions: For EACH ITEM, indicate if it is present or not. Add any clarifying information, then review all information, considering if check indicates a problem or strength and the relationship to and need for care planning. Using the data to validate your decision to proceed or not, document your analysis on the reverse side of this document.

	YES	NO	CLARIFYING INFORMATION
Factors impeding ability to eat			
Chewing problem from oral abscess			
Chewing problem from ill-fitting dentures			
Chewing problems from broken, carious teeth			
Fear of swallowing or choking			
Inability to swallow			
Professional assessment of swallowing problem last 6 to 12 mos.			NA
Reduced ability to feed (e.g., arthritis, contractures, coma, loss of movement, vision problems, cognitive loss, dependence in eating). If yes, indicate why.			NA
Medical causes			
Malignancy and nutritional consequences of chemo/radiation/surgery			
Shortness of breath			
Anemia: paleness of mucous membranes, nailbeds			
Chronic COPD, heart, liver, or kidney disease			
Constipation problems			
Pain			
Drug-induced anorexia. Review meds with pharmacist for potential to alter or decrease appetite, taste, smell, etc.			
Recent acute health problems			
Other causal links			
Dementia, depression, mental retardation, paranoid fears. If yes, identify the problem.			
Behavior problems (e.g., fear, wandering, short attention span, withdrawn, can't or refuses to communicate, uses food as attention getter, etc.). If yes, identify the problem.			
Able to effectively communicate needs/wants (e.g., telling staff there's a problem with food, etc.)			
Dining room conductive to socialization			
Adequate time for feeding and assisting to eat			
Would adaptive feeding equipment enhance ability to feed self?			

Signature/Title of evaluator or person completing RAP _____

The Big Book of Care Plans, Second Edition

RAP Evaluation for Dehydration/Fluid Maintenance

Name _____ Date _____

Directions: For EACH ITEM, indicate if it is present or not. Add any clarifying information, then review all information, considering if check indicates a problem or strength and the relationship to and need for care planning. Using the data to validate your decision to proceed or not, document your analysis on the reverse side of this document.

	YES	NO	CLARIFYING INFORMATION
Moderately or severely impaired decision-making			
Recent unexplained change in mental status or delirious			
Comatose			
Dx of depression, mental retardation, or dementia			
Comprehension or communication problems			
Ability to understand frequently or always impaired			
Ability to be understood by others frequently or always impaired			
Cannot or refuses to communicate			
Body control problems			
Needs extensive assist to transfer and/or unable to move freely about unit			
Difficulty grasping cup. If yes, would adaptive equipment enhance ability?			
Recent decline in ADLs			
Swallowing problems			
Mouth sores or ulcers are present			
Refuses meals, food, or medication			
Able to drink from cup or suck through a straw			
Feeding tube in use			
Dehydration risk factors			
Fluid restrictions ordered			
Fluid restricted by resident or staff to avoid incontinence episodes			
Decrease in thirst perception or unaware of need to take fluids Sad mood, grief, depression			
Excessive sweating, fever or infection			
Vomiting, diarrhea, nausea			
Laxatives, enemas, or diuretics in use			
Urine output exceeds 2000 cc/day			
Urine volume is decreased and concentrated			
Mucous membranes are dry			

Signature/Title of evaluator or person completing RAP _____

RAP Evaluation for Tube Feeding

Name _____ **Date** _____

Directions: For EACH ITEM, indicate if it is present or not. Add any clarifying information, and then review all information. A yes response requires clarification. Document analysis on the reverse side of this document.

	YES	NO	CLARIFYING INFORMATION
Tube feeding is nasogastic			
Tube feeding is other type. If yes, specify type.			
Occurrence of risk factors since tube placement			
Delirium			
Depression			
Agitation or anxiety			
Use of limb restraints to prevent removal of lung aspiration			
Shortness of breath			
Pneumonia, aspiration			
Fever			
Self extubation			
Placement or dislodgment in lung			
Pneumothorax			
Pleural effusion			
Airway obstruction or respiratory distress			
Chest pain			
Loss of heart beat			
Loss of consciousness			
Abdominal distension			
Dehydration			
Nose bleeds			
Fecal impaction or constipation			
Diarrhea			
Care planning considerations			
Are interventions in place to minimize occurrence in all areas checked above?			
Have alternatives been tried or considered to minimize risk?			
Was informed consent obtained? Identify by whom.			
Was right to refuse treatment honored? If no, explain why.			
Is placement temporary? If no, why?			
Expected date of removal is more than one month. If yes, why?			
Alternative to tube feeding has been tried. If no, why?			
Receives oral feedings in addition to tube. If yes, can it be increased?			

Signature/Title of evaluator or person completing RAP _____

 The Big Book of Care Plans, Second Edition

RAP Evaluation for Activities

Name _____ Date _____

Directions: For EACH ITEM, indicate if it is present or not. Add any clarifying information, then review all information, considering if check indicates a problem or strength and the relationship to and need for care planning. Using the data to validate your decision to proceed or not, document your analysis on the reverse side of this document.

	YES	NO	CLARIFYING INFORMATION
Daily routine very different from previous activity in community/NF			
Activities correspond to lifetime values, attitudes, expectations			
Considers leisure activities a waste of time			
Cognitive status is impaired: memory, recall or both			
Has difficulty staying on task or paying attention			
Is able to understand, follow direction			
Is able to be understood			
Exhibits behavior problems			
Sadness or depression is present			
Experiencing a new disability			
Diagnosis or illness necessitates slowing down or limits involvement in activities for which a preference has been stated			
Little time/energy is available after treatment regimen			
Embarrassed or uneasy because of tubes, wheelchair, etc.			
Psychoactive drugs are in use. If yes, indicate impact on participation. Is it better or worse?			
Has resident, staff, or family been overprotective?			
Has staff or family misread seriousness of cognitive or functional decline?			
Are there retained skills, or capacity or desire to learn new activities?			
Is there is a lack of participation in majority of activities for which a preference has been stated?			
Are groups dominated by another resident?			
Is resident shy, unable to make friends?			
Is facility layout conducive to participation? Is resident frustrated by physical features of building?			
Is the resident capable of increased involvement either independently or with a structured program?			
Is it possible to adapt activities for which a preference is known or assumed to meet the functional status of the resident? If not, why?			

Signature/Title of evaluator or person completing RAP _____

Physical Restraint Assessment

Directions: Respond in the most appropriate section for each item listed. Clarify any checks made about compromise. Then consider these factors and complete the analysis at the reverse side. (Can be used as RAP.)

Name _____ Date _____

ASSESSMENT FACTOR	Capable/strength	Compromise/weakness	COMMENTS/CLARIFICATIONS
Able to think/decisions reasonable			
Able to understand			
Able to be understood			
Able to be directed/redirected			
Attention span intact			
Behavior cooperative/manageable			
Mood is pleasant/stable			
Feels safe/secure			
Recognizes/aware of limitations			
Ambulates safely without assistance			
Gait is steady/sure-footed			
Transfers self without aid or assist			
Sitting balance is adequate			
Body movements controlled/voluntary/with no limitation of function			
Vision adequate for safe movement			
Adequate control of bowel/bladder			

MEDICAL STATUS CONCERNS CHECK ALL THAT APPLY.	YES	COMMENTS/CLARIFICATIONS
Major mental illness/disorder		
Huntington's, Multiple Sclerosis, Cerebral Palsy, other neuro/muscular Dx.		
Fresh/healing hip fracture		
Residual weakness from recent major illness or catastrophic event		
Fall last 30–90 days		
Dizziness, vertigo, syncope, or ears ringing		
Orthostatic Hypotension (BP drop 20 pts lie to sit or sit to stand)		
Resists/disrupts needed medical interventions (e.g., TF, IV, O2, catheters, vent, suctioning, wound care, dressings, etc.)		
Takes psychoactive meds		
Other		

Signature/Title of evaluator or person completing RAP _____

The Big Book of Care Plans, Second Edition

Physical Restraint Assessment (cont.)

Analysis and decision-making regarding need for and use of physical restraint

Is the use of a restraint indicated?
❑ NO, other info is required. Comments if any: _____
❑ YES. Use the information on the reverse side to assist in summarizing your rationale for use.

Specific medical circumstance/need: _____
_____
_____

Other interventions tried and/or ruled out or underway: _____
_____
_____

How will restraint assist in optimizing physical and psychosocial functioning?
_____
_____

Key risk factors associated with use for this resident: Refer to care plan for interventions.
_____

❑ Entrapment/strangulation ❑ Constipation ❑ Pressure Ulcer ❑ Falls
❑ Reduced/loss of mobility ❑ Muscle wasting ❑ Contractures ❑ Isolation
❑ Loss of appetite/weight ❑ Dehydration ❑ Loss of self esteem ❑ Increased behavior
❑ Withdraw ❑ Depression ❑ Increased confusion ❑ Incontinence/increased incontinence
❑ Edema ❑ Infections ❑ Dehydration
Other _____

Type of restraint	Circumstances for use	Duration of application

- All restraints are to be checked every 30 minutes for restrictions and released every two hours, and resident exercised.
- Side Rails used as restraints require checking the resident to ensure safety every _____ minutes/hours as determined by the results of the assessment.

Plan for progressive removal to be initiated   ❑ Immediately   ❑ 1 to 2 weeks   ❑ 30 days   Refer to care plan.

❑ Not anticipated, restraint is least restrictive and used for least amount of time possible, no other interventions are feasible, continued care planning for prevention of risk will be done.

❑ Resident   ❑ Family   ❑ Guardian informed and agrees to plan. These parties sign below.

_____   Date _____
_____   Date _____
_____   Date _____

Signature/Title of evaluator or person completing RAP _____

Urinary Incontinence RAP

Name	Date	Evaluator
❏ High risk: Dependent mob/severe cognitive impairment	❏ Low risk: all other incontinent residents	

Directions: Identify key issues and strengths. This becomes your basis for proceeding or not proceeding to care plans.

Considerations	Yes	No	Clarifications and comments
Conditions present Urinary tract infection ruled out ❏ U/A done ❏ C&S done ❏ Pain with urination			
Bowel impaction ruled out ❏ Rectal exam done and negative			
Delirium present (acute confusion)			
Exhibits signs of depression (noted on MDS)			
Concurrent Medical Problems ❏ Diabetes ❏ High blood glucose ❏ Edema ❏ CHF ❏ CVA ❏ Parkinson's ❏ Recurrent UTI ❏ Fecal impaction			
Dementia ❏ No awareness of urges ❏ Some awareness			
❏ Can respond to urges ❏ Can cooperate			
Cancer ❏ Bladder ❏ Prostate ❏ Brain ❏ Spine			
Environment/Functional Status Requires help to transfer			
Requires help for locomotion			
Distance problems getting to toilet			
Access problems to toilet			
Able to find the toilet			
❏ Can manage clothing ❏ Can wipe self			
Restraints and/or side rails used			
Medications ❏ Diuretics output ❏ > 1 liter/day ❏ < 1 liter/day			
❏ Disopyramide ❏ Antispasmodics			
❏ Sympathomimetics ❏ Beta blockers			
❏ Calcium channel blockers ❏ Parkinson med			
❏ Antipsychotic ❏ Antianxiety/hypnotic			
❏ Antidepressants ❏ Narcotics			
Bladder Tracking Results ❏ Pattern to voiding ❏ No pattern established			
Suspected Type of Incontinence ❏ Stress ❏ Urge ❏ Overflow/obstruction ❏ Functional ❏ Neurogenic			

Signature/Title of evaluator or person completing RAP _____

RAP Review: Indwelling Catheters

Name _____ Date _____

Directions: Respond to each guideline listed. Complete comment/clarification section as needed and directed.

RAP Guidelines	YES	NO	N/A	Comments/clarifications
Has assessment been made for continuing need within past three to six months by urologist?				
Has there been a trial without the catheter? *If yes note results; if no indicate why not and plan.*				
Have there been other assessments to rule out continuing need? *If so, what?*				
Is it the resident's desire or preference to have catheter? *If so, why?*				
If yes, have alternatives been discussed if not contraindicated?				
Does the resident understand the risk associated with use of catheter?				
Is placement short term? Explain.				
Criteria for Use (If none are present contact physician and request further evaluation.)				
Validating diagnosis or reason for use documented?				
Terminal illness?				
Stage 3 or 4 pressure ulcer?				
Obesity prevents adequate toileting/skin care.				
Untreatable urinary blockage? *(Inoperable related to diagnosis or general medical condition.)*				
Catheter required to measure accurate output? If yes, why?				
Problem Factors for Consideration ✔ If yes to any of the following and NO criteria for use established, request trial without catheter. ✔ If yes to any of the following with yes to any criteria for use, explore additional interventions/needs.				
Treated for UTI in the absence of symptoms.				
Treated for UTI with active symptoms of infection (e.g., fever, chills, change in sensorium).				
Fluid intake less than 500 cc per day.				
Irrigation for other than urinary blockage.				
Hx of hospitalization for septicemia, bacteria, pyelonephritis.				
Catheter tube placement problem (e.g., kinking, pressure on tubing, not hung below level of bladder, etc.)				
Tube anchoring system used				

Signature/Title of evaluator or person completing RAP _____

Place this form on the back of each RAP with exception of drug and restraint RAPs.

RAP Evaluation and Analysis For _____ **Date** _____
Identify RAP

MDS 2.0 Triggering Items

Analysis for care planning
Refer to related/linked RAPs _____ and/or:

Key issues

_____
_____
_____

Strengths

_____
_____
_____

Risk factors/potential complications

_____
_____
_____

Care planning decision: ❏ Proceed   ❏ Do not proceed

Potential for improvement: ❏ Improve current status   ❏ Maintain   ❏ Slow decline   ❏ Minimize/prevent complications

Referrals made to: ❏ Nursing   ❏ Social service   ❏ Dietary   ❏ Activities
                            ❏ Therapy   ❏ Physician   ❏ Other _____

Signature/title of person completing RAP analysis: _____

Annual analysis upgrade if triggered   **Date** _____

Signature/Title of evaluator or person completing RAP _____

Fall Risk Assessment and RAP Review

Name _____ Date _____

Directions: Evaluate each item, circling applicable responses. Consider update weekly x 4 for new admissions, and quarterly and as needed thereafter.

Risk Factors Review	Status of Indicators	Date	Date	Date	Date
Mental status	Impaired short-term memory	1	1	1	1
	No recall	2	2	2	2
	Mental status varies	3	3	3	3
Ambulation/bed mobility	Dependent on others	1	1	1	1
	Supervision with assistive devices	2	2	2	2
	Physical support required/Independent unaware of safety needs	3	3	3	3
Continence	Occ. incont urine 2+/wk; bowel 2–3/wk	1	1	1	1
	Freq. incont. urine daily; bowel 2–3/wk	2	2	2	2
	Always incont. Bowel and bladder	3	3	3	3
Vision/sensory	Needs glasses to see adequately	1	1	1	1
	Vision poor with/without glasses or blind	2	2	2	2
	Vision poor and lacks sensation feet/hands	3	3	3	3
Fluid intake	Unaware of thirst, needs assist to drink	1	1	1	1
	Drinks fluids only at meal time	2	2	2	2
	Does not drink or resist drinking	3	3	3	3
Edema	Present	3	3	3	3
Meds predisposing falls ❑ Antipsychotic ❑ Antianxiety ❑ Hypnotic ❑ Pain ❑ Antihistamine ❑ Diuretic ❑ Cardiovascular	Daily or change in dose last 30 days	1	1	1	1
	More than daily, no falls last 30 days	2	2	2	2
	Daily or more, falls last 30 days	3	3	3	3
Predisposing factors ❑ Anemia ❑ Arthritis ❑ CA ❑ COPD ❑ CVA ❑ DM ❑ MS ❑ Falls > 30days ❑ Fractures ❑ Hemi/quad ❑ Vascular disease	One or two present	1	1	1	1
	Three or four present	2	2	2	2
	Five or more and/or terminal condition	3	3	3	3
Additional key factors ❑ Physical restraint ❑ Side rails ❑ Cane/walker ❑ G/C tray ❑ W/C ❑ Belt/lap buddy	One present	1	1	1	1
	Two or three present	2	2	2	2
	Four or more and/or terminal condition	3	3	3	3
Total score: 10 or higher indicates risk for falls is present.					
Reviewer _____					

Skin Risk Assessment and RAP Review

Name _____ Date _____

Directions: Circle the score next to the most appropriate indicator in each section, check all areas that are present in left hand column.

Review Area	Status of Indicator	Date	Date	Date	Date
Mental status	Alert and oriented x 3	0	0	0	0
	Lethargic, slow to respond	1	1	1	1
	Only responds to verbal or painful stimuli	2	2	2	2
	Unresponsive	3	3	3	3
Ambulation/bed mobility	Independent	0	0	0	0
	Limited assistance	1	1	1	1
	Extensive assistance or chairfast	2	2	2	2
	Totally dependent or bedfast	3	3	3	3
Continence	Control of bowel and bladder	0	0	0	0
	Occ. incont urine 2+/wk; bowel 2–3/wk	1	1	1	1
	Freq. incont. urine daily; bowel 2–3/wk	2	2	2	2
	Always incont. bowel and bladder	3	3	3	3
Nutrition/weight	Eats everything offered or weight heavy for size	0	0	0	0
	Eats 75–100% or weight appears adequate for size	1	1	1	1
	Eats 50–75% or appears below weight for size	2	2	2	2
	Eats less than 25% or appears thin and emaciated	3	3	3	3
Fluid intake	Liberal with meals and throughout day	0	0	0	0
	Drinks fluids only at meal time	1	1	1	1
	Drinks with assistance or unaware of thirst	2	2	2	2
	Does not drink or resists drinking	3	3	3	3
Edema	Present	3	3	3	3
Medications/treatment ❑ Analgesics ❑ Psychoactive Drug(s) ❑ Steroids ❑ Dialysis ❑ Chemo ❑ Radiation ❑ IV med	None	0	0	0	0
	One to two present	1	1	1	1
	Three present	2	2	2	2
	Four or more or terminal prognosis	3	3	3	3
Predisposing factors ❑ Anemia ❑ Arthritis ❑ CA ❑ COPD ❑ CVA ❑ DM ❑ MS ❑ Pain ❑ Falls > 30 days ❑ Fractures ❑ Hemi/quad ❑ Hx/presence ulcers any type ❑ Vascular diagnosis	None	0	0	0	0
	One or two present	1	1	1	1
	Three or four present	2	2	2	2
	Five or more present and/or terminal condition	3	3	3	3
Additional key factors ❑ Physical restraints ❑ Side rails ❑ Skin desensitized to pain ❑ Impaired cognition ❑ Depressed/withdrawn	None	0	0	0	0
	One present	1	1	1	1
	Two or three present	2	2	2	2
	Four or more present and/or terminal condition	3	3	3	3
Total score of 8 or more indicates need for care planning.					
Name/initials of reviewer _____					

The Big Book of Care Plans, Second Edition

Activity Assessment and RAP Review

Name _____ DOB _____

Review date _____ Type of Review: ❑ Adm.   ❑ Annual   ❑ Sig. change   ❑ Other

Interview conducted with: ❑ Resident   ❑ Family   ❑ Both   ❑ Sig. other   ❑ None, reason _____

History and Lifestyle

Religion: ❑ Catholic   ❑ Protestant _____   ❑ Jewish   ❑ Other _____

❑ Practicing, finds strength in faith   ❑ Non-practicing   ❑ Wants to resume practicing   ❑ Not interested in practicing

Political involvement: ❑ No   ❑ Yes   Desire to vote: ❑ No   ❑ Yes

Comments: _____

Type of work	
Clubs or organizations	
Pets	
Hobbies	
Fondest memories	
Achievements, things most proud of	
Usual routine prior to entry to NF	❑ Stays up after 9 pm ❑ Naps regularly during day (> 1hr) ❑ Goes out 1+day/wk ❑ Uses tobacco daily ❑ Stays busy with hobbies, reading, or fixed routine ❑ Spends most time alone or watching TV

Check all activity interest and indicate   **P** = Past   **C** = Current   **L** = Would like to learn/do

Activity preferences	P	C	L	Comments/clarifications/specifics
Arts and crafts				
Games/cards				
Exercise				
Sports				
Music				
Reading/writing				
Talking/conversing				
Helping others				
Gardening/plants				
Spiritual/religious				
Being outside				
Watching TV				
Sewing				
Clubs				
Other				

Daily routine (Include both structured and non-structured things the resident does daily or almost daily)

Use of tobacco products at least daily ❑ No   ❑ Yes   Use of alcoholic beverages at least weekly ❑ No   ❑ Yes

Coffee/tea and paper in morning: ❑ No   ❑ Yes   Usual time _____

❑ Radio station _____   ❑ TV programs _____

Preferred settings for activities   Check all that apply.

❑ Own room   ❑ Day/activity room   ❑ Inside facility/off unit   ❑ Outside facility   ❑ Outdoors

AVERAGE TIME SPENT Structured/scheduled activities ❑ None   ❑ < 1/3   ❑ 1/3 to 2/3   ❑ > 2/3

AVERAGE TIME SPENT pursuing interest independently ❑ None   ❑ < 1/3   ❑ 1/3 to 2/3   ❑ > 2/3

Most active time of day: ❑ Morning   ❑ Afternoon   ❑ Evenings

Usual rising time _____   Naps: ❑ No ❑ Yes, time _____   Usual bedtime _____   Wakes during night ❑ No ❑ Yes

Activities prior to going to bed _____

_____

Activity Assessment and RAP Review (cont.)

RAP Guidlines and Potential Factors Affecting Participation

Name _____

Directions: Check all that apply, then consider their impact and relationship to care planning.

Physical Factors to Consider
Status over past 90 days or since last assessment: ❑ Unchanged   ❑ Improved   ❑ Deteriorated

❑ Acute health problems   ❑ Recently recovered acute health problems   ❑ Health status varies over day   ❑ Tires easily   ❑ Motor agitation or restlessness
❑ Lacks energy/drive   ❑ Incontinent bowel/bladder   ❑ Pain limits/prevents participation   ❑ Physical restraints used   ❑ Psychoactive drugs used
❑ Treatments leave little energy for activities   ❑ Physical layout impedes involvement/participation   ❑ Vision impaired, not corrected with glasses
❑ Speech slurred, hard to understand or absent

_____
_____
_____
_____

Cognitive Factors to Consider
Cognition over past 90 days or since last assessment: ❑ Unchanged   ❑ Improved   ❑ Deteriorated

❑ Short-term memory impaired   ❑ Long-term memory impaired   ❑ Problems with recall   ❑ Attention span short   ❑ Problems understanding
❑ Problems being understood   ❑ Can't/won't engage in conversation   ❑ Conversation lacks substance   ❑ Can't initiate activity

_____
_____
_____
_____

Social/Spiritual/Emotional Factors to Consider
Mood/Behavior over past 90 days or since last assessment: ❑ Unchanged   ❑ Improved   ❑ Deteriorated

❑ Seems sad or depressed   ❑ Makes frequent negative comments   ❑ Not easily cheered   ❑ Angry, Irritable   ❑ Agitated with increased stimulation
❑ Exhibits repetitive behaviors   ❑ Socially inappropriate   ❑ Dominates others   ❑ Verbally abusive   ❑ Physically aggressive/abusive to residents/staff
❑ Wanders, has difficulty sitting still   ❑ Shy, unable to make friends   ❑ Lonely, lacks familiar contact
❑ Embarrassed by tubes, equipment, personal appearance   ❑ Comfortable with status quo, unwilling to make changes or learn new things of interest
❑ Doesn't participate in activities stated of interest

_____
_____
_____
_____

Activity Assessment and RAP Review (cont.)

Activity Care Planning Considerations

Name _____

Strengths to Draw On

❑ Health status is stable   ❑ Energetic, has stamina   ❑ Independent in mobility   ❑ Continent of B&B   ❑ Readily engages in activities
❑ Enjoys physical activity/exercise   ❑ Enjoys passive act.   ❑ Able to think and make decisions   ❑ Readily engages in conversation   ❑ Follows instructions
❑ Able to be redirecte   ❑ Adjusts easily to change   ❑ At ease interacting with others   ❑ At ease doing planned activities   ❑ Establishes own goals
❑ Finds strength in faith   ❑ Strong identification with past roles   ❑ Seems happy, content   ❑ Pleasant to others   ❑ Assumes leadership
❑ Pursues involvement/tries new things   ❑ Initiates activities on own   ❑ Frequent contact with family, friends

Projected Level of Participation

❑ Active involvement in structured program   ❑ Passive involvement in structured program   ❑ Both active and passive participation
❑ In-room self-initiated activities by choice and lifestyle. Room visits (freq.____)   ❑ In-room staff-supported activities/resident choice/lifestyle or medical necessity.
❑ 1-to-1 programming R/T functional status/problems

Care Planning Decision

❑ **Do not proceed**, resident's medical condition and/or treatment regimen prohibits involvement or participation.
  ❑ Reading   ❑ Radio   ❑ TV   is/are only diversion(s) indicated or desired.

❑ **Proceed to care planning using activities as an area of strength.** Resident is self-initiating, presents little to no risk or is highly involved in current programs. Activity strengths will be incorporated as appropriate in other problem/need areas of care plan.

❑ **Proceed to care planning for possible adverse effects** related to compromised medical condition and/or inability to be involved or participate in activities without support/assistance.

❑ Proceed to care plan as inactivity or current program plans are/may be causing or contributing to other problems.

❑ Proceed to care planning. Requires teaching related to _____.

Types of Programs Resident May Benefit From

Promotion/maintenance of   ❑ Physical functioning   ❑ Psychosocial functioning   ❑ Spiritual needs

❑ Socialization   ❑ Solace: comfort, distraction   ❑ Empowerment   ❑ Cognitive functioning   ❑ Sensory stimulation   ❑ Discharge preparation
❑ Education/training (e.g., leisure activities)   ❑ Community outreach programs (e.g., BVR, MRDD)

Additional Remarks

_____
_____
_____
_____
_____
_____

Activity Assessment and RAP Review (cont.)

Activity Quarterly and Periodic Assessment

Name _____ Date _____

Type of review ❏ 5-day ❏ 14-day ❏ 30-day ❏ 60-day ❏ 90-day

Responses should encompass the time frame from last assessment completed. If significant deviation from usual/average occurs within seven days of MDS reference date, clarify in comments section.

COGNITION   ❏ Unchanged   ❏ Improved   ❏ Deteriorated

COMMUNICATION ❏ Unchanged   ❏ Improved   ❏ Deteriorated

❏ Alert and oriented   ❏ At ease interacting with others   ❏ At ease doing planned activities   ❏ Chooses activities to do

❏ Confused, but able to be directed ❏ Confused, difficult/unable to engage ❏ Short-term memory impaired   ❏ Long-term memory impaired

❏ Problems with recall   ❏ Attention span short   ❏ Problems understanding   ❏ Problems being understood

❏ Can't/won't engage in conversation ❏ Conversation lacks substance   ❏ Can't initiate activity

_____

_____

_____

_____

MOOD   ❏ Unchanged   ❏ Improved   ❏ Deteriorated

BEHAVIOR   ❏ Unchanged   ❏ Improved   ❏ Deteriorated

Consider factors as they relate to activity involvement and activity program.

❏ Pleasant/happy/content   ❏ Enjoys structured activities   ❏ Enjoys activities of own choosing   ❏ Seems sad/unhappy

❏ Easily cheered up   ❏ Voices negative comments a lot   ❏ Physically hits self or others   ❏ Wanders in and out of activities

❏ Socially inappropriate behavior   ❏ Stubborn, resistive, refuses to cooperate ❏ Screams/curses/threatens others

_____

_____

_____

_____

PHYSICAL RESTRAINTS/SIDE RAILS ❏ Not used ❏ In use, ACT status declined? ❏ NO ❏ YES

PSYCHOACTIVE DRUGS   ❏ Not used ❏ In use, ACT status declined? ❏ NO ❏ YES

If in use and/or status decline explain and indicate effect on activities:

_____

_____

_____

_____

_____

 The Big Book of Care Plans, Second Edition

Activity Assessment and RAP Review (cont.)

Activity Quarterly and Periodic Assessment (cont.)

TIME AWAKE AND AVAILABLE for activity pursuits ❑ None ❑ Morning ❑ Afternoon ❑ Evening
If naps/dozes greater than one hour in any time period do not check the box.

AVERAGE TIME SPENT structured/scheduled activities ❑ None ❑ < 1/3 ❑ 1/3 to 2/3 ❑ > 2/3

AVERAGE TIME SPENT pursuing interests independently ❑ None ❑ < 1/3 ❑ 1/3 to 2/3 ❑ > 2/3
INITIATIVE ❑ Independent ❑ Needs prompts/encouragement ❑ Will not initiate ❑ Cannot initiate

PARTICIPATION HAS ❑ Remained the same ❑ Improved ❑ Declined
PREFERRED SETTING ❑ Own room ❑ Day/activity room ❑ Inside NF/off unit ❑ Outside

PREFERS CHANGE IN ACTIVITIES ❑ None ❑ Slight ❑ Major

Activity care planning ❑ Remains appropriate ❑ Will be initiated and/or modified

Additional comments

_____
_____
_____
_____
_____
_____
_____
_____
_____
_____
_____
_____
_____
_____
_____
_____
_____
_____
_____
_____
_____

Signature/title _____

Social Service History

Name _____ DOB _____

To be completed on admission only.   **Interview conducted with:** ❑ Resident   ❑ Family   ❑ Both   ❑ Neither

Updates can be made on a trailer sheet or on progress notes

I. Lifestyle and history

Birthplace: _____   **Zip code of primary residence:** _____

Admitted from

❑ Private home/apt.   ❑ Lived with family/significant other   ❑ With home health   ❑ Without home health

❑ Other facility   ❑ Lived alone   ❑ Board and care home/assisted living/group home

❑ Nursing home   ❑ MR/DD unit   ❑ MH/psychiatric hospital   ❑ Acute care hospital

❑ Rehabilitative hospital   ❑ Other _____

Resident participated in decision to enter nursing home? ❑ Yes   ❑ No, explain response.

Explain reason for admission and describe events leading up to placement

_____

_____

_____

Residential history past five years

❑ None   ❑ Prior stay in this NF   ❑ Prior stay another NF   ❑ Other residential facility   ❑ MH/Psych setting   ❑ MR/DD setting

II. Ethnic background

❑ Caucasian   ❑ Black, not of Hispanic origin   ❑ Hispanic   ❑ American Indian/Alaskan Native   ❑ Asian Pacific Islander

❑ Other _____   Primary language spoken _____

III. Family history

Parents' names: _____

Number of brothers: _____   Sisters: _____   All living? ❑ Yes ❑ No

Names: _____

Family and marriage: ❑ Single   ❑ Alternative lifestyle   ❑ Married   ❑ Widowed   ❑ Divorced

Number of times married: _____   divorced: _____   widowed: _____   Spouse's name: _____

Children: ❑ No ❑ Yes # Boys: _____   # Girls: _____   All living? ❑ Yes ❑ No

Names: _____

Daily contact with family, friends? ❑ Yes ❑ No

Family situation and relationships; nature of relationships, significant impacting factors

_____

_____

IV. General personality traits *(If comatose, skip to Section IX)*

❑ Easygoing   ❑ Enjoys attention   ❑ Enjoys listening to others/being needed   ❑ Thoughtful and deliberate   ❑ Dominant   ❑ Task oriented

❑ Impulsive   ❑ Feelings easily hurt   ❑ Infrequently shows feelings   ❑ Other: _____

Typical response in stressful situations:

❑ Withdrawn   ❑ Passive/aggressive   ❑ Aggressive towards others   ❑ Rant, rave, throw a "temper tantrum" (agrees and then doesn't comply)

Social Service History (cont.)

V. Spiritual life

❑ Catholic ❑ Jewish ❑ Protestant, denomination: _____ ❑ Other: _____
❑ Finds strength in faith ❑ Attends religious services ❑ Does not attend
Comments: _____

VI. Community life

Political involvement? ❑ No ❑ Yes **Active voter?** ❑ No ❑ Yes ❑ Wants to be
Cultural and social interest: _____
_____

VII. Education

❑ No school ❑ 8th grade or less ❑ Grade 9–11 ❑ High school graduate ❑ Tech school ❑ Some college ❑ Bachelor degree
❑ Graduate degree ❑ Other training: _____

VIII. Occupational background   Date of retirement_____

❑ Business ❑ Industrial ❑ Healthcare ❑ Domestic ❑ Laborer ❑ Construction ❑ Self Employed ❑ Manager
❑ Teacher ❑ Secretary ❑ Housewife ❑ Salesperson ❑ Other _____
Military Service, branch: _____
Specific Occupation: _____

IX. Responsibility

❑ Self ❑ Family member ❑ Legal guardian ❑ Other legal oversight ❑ Durable power of attorney for healthcare ❑ Finances

X. Advanced care directives

❑ None in place ❑ No desire to put in place ❑ Desires assistance to develop ❑ Living will ❑ DNR ❑ Do not hospitalize
❑ Documents in medical record ❑ Organ donor ❑ Request autopsy ❑ Feeding restrictions ❑ Medication/treatment restrictions
❑ Durable power of attorney for healthcare ❑ Other _____

XI. Financial resources

❑ Private pay ❑ Private ❑ Medicare ❑ Medicaid ❑ VA ❑ Champus ❑ Other: _____

XII. Discharge planning

Discharge is anticipated: ❑ Not anticipated ❑ Within 30 days ❑ Within 31–90 days
❑ Other _____

Wants to return to community: ❑ No ❑ Yes **Support person in agreement:** ❑ Yes ❑ No
Discharge possibilities: ❑ None ❑ Lesser care setting ❑ Home ❑ Other _____
Address impact if not feasible/realistic.

Signature/title of evaluator _____

Social Service Assessment and RAP Review: Cognition, Mood, Behavior, and Well Being

Name _____ Date _____

Type of Review: ❑ Admission   ❑ Annual   ❑ Significant Change   ❑ Other _____

Interview Conducted with: ❑ Resident   ❑ Family   ❑ Both   ❑ Sig. Other   ❑ None, reason _____

Comatose? ❑ No   ❑ Yes, STOP HERE. Refer to Social History

I. Potential Problems, Complications, and Adjustment Concerns

Recent Changes in Environment

❑ Admitted to nursing facility   ❑ Change in room/mate   ❑ Loss of family/friend   ❑ Staff changes   ❑ Usual habits disrupted

❑ Unable to accommodate preferences   ❑ Anger over placement   ❑ Voices/acts out wanting to leave   ❑ Difficulty adjusting to changes in routine

❑ Difficulty adjusting to placement   ❑ Perceives that daily routine is very different from prior pattern

Financial Status

❑ Recently altered   ❑ Fear of/loss of funds   ❑ No control of funds   ❑ Welfare application   ❑ Other

Relationship Issues

❑ Expresses conflict/anger with family/friends   ❑ Absence of personal contact with family/friends   ❑ Recent loss of close family/friend

❑ Covert/open conflict or repeated criticism of staff   ❑ Unhappy with room/mate/other residents   ❑ Other: _____

Physical Status

❑ Changes in body image or physical functioning   ❑ Presence of or complaints of pain

❑ New or worsening condition/illness (e.g., cancer, diabetes, CHF, stroke)

Impact/Risk on psychosocial status

❑ None   ❑ Frustration   ❑ Anxiety   ❑ Verbal abuse   ❑ Physical Abuse   ❑ Depressed Mood   ❑ Agitation

❑ Withdrawal   ❑ Wandering/Elopement

_____

_____

II. Cognitive Patterns   Check all that apply.

Short-Term Memory intact (Can remember longer than 5 minutes)?   ❑ Yes   ❑ No

Long-Term Memory intact (Can recall long-past events)?   ❑ Yes   ❑ No

Memory/Recall

❑ Current season   ❑ Location of room   ❑ That in a nursing facility   ❑ Staff names/faces   ❑ None of these

❑ Can't distinguish belongings/room from others   ❑ Can't recognize family/friends

Oriented to: ❑ Time of day   ❑ Day of week   ❑ Month of year   ❑ Year   ❑ None of these

Ability to Learn/Remember: ❑ No, cannot learn/remember   ❑ Yes, on own   ❑ With reinforcement

Attention span: ❑ Reasonable   ❑ Short

Able to be redirected? ❑ Yes   ❑ With difficulty   ❑ No

_____

_____

Ability to Think AND Make Decisions

❑ Decisions are consistent and reasonable   ❑ Difficulty making decisions in new situations   ❑ Altered perception

❑ Poor decisions, needs cues/supervision   ❑ Never/rarely makes decisions   ❑ Easily distracted   ❑ Episodes of disorganized speech

❑ Periods of restlessness   ❑ Periods of lethargy   ❑ Mental status varies over the day

❑ Different from usual functioning/resident/family or caregivers

          The Big Book of Care Plans, Second Edition

Social Service Assessment and RAP Review: Cognition, Mood, Behavior, and Well Being (cont.)

Difficulty Occurred ❑ NA ❑ last 7 days ❑ last 30 days ❑ longer

Problems with decision-making seem related to

❑ NA ❑ Personality, life-long habit ❑ Cognitive loss ❑ Depression, sad mood, or apathy ❑ Combination of all of these ❑ Unknown or unsure

Environmental Stimuli

❑ Responds appropriately ❑ Disturbed by groups of people, activities, etc. ❑ Seems bored, disengaged
❑ Misinterprets voices, sounds, radio, TV, pictures, objects, etc.

Cognitive Status past 90 days or since last assessment: ❑ Unchanged ❑ Improved ❑ Deteriorated

Impact/Risk of areas noted on psychosocial status: ❑ None ❑ Frustration ❑ Anxiety ❑ Verbal abuse ❑ Physical Abuse
❑ Depressed Mood ❑ Agitation ❑ Withdrawal ❑ Wandering/Elopement

Analysis, including suspected cause of any status deterioration: _____
_____

III. Communication Patterns

Hearing

❑ Hears normal talk, TV, phone ❑ Minimal difficulty ❑ Speaker must adjust tonal quality/speak distinctly
❑ Highly impaired, absence of useful hearing ❑ Has a hearing aid ❑ Uses aid
❑ Does not use, reason: _____
Special needs related to hearing aid: _____

Hearing evaluation conducted past year? ❑ Yes ❑ No **Indicated?** ❑ Yes ❑ No
Resources available? ❑ Yes ❑ No

Modes of Expression
❑ Speech ❑ Lip reads ❑ Writes to clarify needs ❑ Sign language/Braille ❑ Signs/gestures/sounds ❑ Communication board
❑ Other _____ ❑ None of these ❑ Speech clear ❑ Speech unclear ❑ No speech
Speech evaluation done? ❑ Yes ❑ No
Vision: ❑ Adequate to see others ❑ Adequate to read ❑ Inadequate or none
Ability to understand: ❑ Always ❑ Usually ❑ Sometimes ❑ Never/Almost never
Ability to be understood: ❑ Always ❑ Usually ❑ Sometimes ❑ Never/Almost never
Impact/Risk on psychosocial status: ❑ None ❑ Frustration ❑ Anxiety ❑ Verbal abuse ❑ Wandering/Elopement ❑ Depressed Mood
❑ Agitation ❑ Withdrawal ❑ Physical Abuse
Communication past 90 days or since last assessment: ❑ Unchanged ❑ Improved ❑ Deteriorated
_____
_____

IV. Mood AND Well Being Patterns

GENERAL WELL BEING

❑ At ease interacting with others ❑ At ease doing planned activities ❑ Accepts invitations to groups ❑ At ease doing self-initiated activities
❑ Pursues involvement in NF ❑ Establishes own goals ❑ Expresses feelings ❑ Makes needs known
❑ Seems content, accepting of placement ❑ Strong ID with past roles
Status past 90 days or since last assessment: ❑ Unchanged ❑ Improved ❑ Deteriorated

Social Service Assessment and RAP Review: Cognition, Mood, Behavior, and Well Being (cont.)

VERBAL EXPRESSIONS OF DISTRESS

❏ Negative self statements   ❏ Repetitive Questions   ❏ Repetitive Verbalization   ❏ Persistent anger   ❏ Self deprecation

❏ Expression of unreal fears   ❏ Statements that something bad is about to happen   ❏ Repetitive health complaints

❏ Repetitive complaints/concerns   ❏ Repetitive movements   ❏ Suicidal thoughts

SLEEP CYCLE

❏ Unpleasant mood in morning   ❏ Insomnia/Changes in sleep pattern   ❏ Wakes to toilet

❏ Routinely sleeps through night   ❏ Routinely does not sleep through night

SADNESS, APATHY, LOSS OF INTEREST

❏ Crying/tearful   ❏ Sad/pained/worried facial expression   ❏ Withdrawn from activities   ❏ Reduced social interaction   ❏ Takes little/no initiative

Mood Status past 90 days or since last assessment: ❏ Unchanged   ❏ Improved   ❏ Deteriorated

❏ Mood indicators not present or easily altered

❏ Mood indicators not easily altered

IMPACT/RISK OF AREAS NOTED ON PSYCHOSOCIAL STATUS:

❏ None   ❏ Frustration   ❏ Anxiety   ❏ Verbal Abuse   ❏ Physical Abuse   ❏ Agitation   ❏ Wandering/Elopement

❏ Withdrawal   ❏ Depressed Mood

Analysis, including suspected cause of any status deterioration:

_____

_____

_____

V. Physical Restraints AND Devices   ❏ NA Skip to next section.

Use prevents from coming and going freely of own accord or touching one part to another? ❏ NO   ❏ YES

Type of device being used: ❏ Side rails   ❏ Geri-chair   ❏ Jacket   ❏ Belt   ❏ Recliner   ❏ Other

Stated reason for use: ❏ Treat medical symptoms   ❏ Behavior management   ❏ Supportive device

Informed consent obtained? ❏ No, reason: _____   ❏ Yes, who: _____

Non-medical interventions tried prior to use? ❏ Yes   ❏ No, reason: _____

Reduction/elimination underway or indicated? ❏ Yes   ❏ No, reason: _____

_____

_____

_____

VI. Psychoactive Medication   ❏ NA Skip to next section.

Type Drug: ❏ Antipsychotic   ❏ Long-acting anti-anxiety   ❏ Short-acting anti-anxiety   ❏ Antidepressant   ❏ Hypnotic   ❏ Other

❏ Long-standing use prior to admission   ❏ Ordered on admission   ❏ Ordered following admission

Name of drug: _____   **Reason for use:** _____

Informed consent obtained? ❏ No, reason: _____   ❏ Yes, who: _____

Non-medical interventions tried prior to use ❏ Yes   ❏ No, reason: _____

Is reduction/elimination underway or indicated ❏ Yes   ❏ No, reason: _____

_____

_____

_____

 The Big Book of Care Plans, Second Edition

Social Service Assessment and RAP Review: Cognition, Mood, Behavior, and Well Being (cont.)

VII. Behavior Patterns

Wanders

Occurrence: ❏ Never/rarely ❏ 1–3 days/wk ❏ 4–6 days/wk ❏ Daily or more

❏ Halls, public areas ❏ In and out of resident rooms ❏ Attempts to wander outside ❏ Other

Verbally Abusive

Occurrence: ❏ Never/rarely ❏ 1–3 days/wk ❏ 4–6 days/wk ❏ Daily or more

❏ During care times ❏ In response to environmental factors real or perceived ❏ When angry

❏ As a lifestyle/personality trait ❏ No clear precipitant

Physically Abusive

Occurrence: ❏ Never/rarely ❏ 1–3 days/wk ❏ 4–6 days/wk ❏ Daily or more

❏ During care times ❏ In response to environmental factors real or perceived ❏ When angry

❏ As a lifestyle/personality trait ❏ No clear precipitant

Socially Inappropriate/Disruptive

❏ Never/rarely ❏ 1–3 days/wk ❏ 4–6 days/wk ❏ Daily or more

❏ Disruptive sounds/noises ❏ Screaming ❏ Self-abusive acts ❏ Sexual behavior in public ❏ Disrobing in public

❏ Smears/hoards/throws feces, food ❏ Rummages through others' belongings ❏ Other _____

Resistive to care efforts

Occurrence: ❏ Never/rarely ❏ 1–3 days/wk ❏ 4–6 days/wk ❏ Daily or more

❏ Bathing ❏ Dressing ❏ Grooming ❏ Oral care ❏ Eating ❏ Medical Treatments ❏ Restorative/ Rehab care

❏ Medication administration ❏ Other _____

BEHAVIOR PAST 90 DAYS OR SINCE LAST ASSESSMENT: ❏ Unchanged ❏ Improved ❏ Deteriorated

❏ Behaviors not present or easily altered

❏ Behavior present and not easily altered

Suspected cause for behavior problems:

❏ Pain/Discomfort ❏ Illness acute or chronic ❏ Cognitive compromise ❏ Misinterpretation of events ❏ Staff approach

❏ Depression, sad mood ❏ Anger at situation ❏ Attempt to express unmet need ❏ Overstimulation ❏ Understimulation

❏ Physical restraints ❏ Medication ❏ Other

Analysis, including suspected cause of any status deterioration.

_____

_____

_____

VIII. Discharge Planning

Discharge is anticipated: ❏ Not anticipated ❏ Within 30 days ❏ Within 31–90 days ❏ Other

Discharge possibilities: ❏ Lesser care setting ❏ Home ❏ Other

Wants to return to community? ❏ Yes ❏ No **Support person in agreement?** ❏ Yes ❏ No

Address impact if not feasible/realistic.

_____

_____

_____

Social Service Assessment and RAP Review: Cognition, Mood, Behavior, and Well Being (cont.)

Intervention programs/Referrals for mood, behavior and cognitive loss

May Benefit From

Date Initiated if in Progress

❑ Special behavior symptom evaluation program ❑ _____

❑ Group therapy (support, psychodynamic, medical issues, etc) ❑ _____

❑ Resident-specific environmental changes to address mood/behavior pattern ❑ _____

❑ Reorientation ❑ _____

❑ Remotivation ❑ _____

❑ Socialization ❑ _____

❑ Individual counseling ❑ _____

❑ Behavior management program ❑ _____

❑ Evaluation by mental health specialist ❑ _____

❑ Psychiatrist ❑ Psychologist ❑ Other licensed MH specialist ❑ _____

❑ Discharge preparation ❑ _____

❑ Education/training ❑ _____

❑ Community outreach programs (e.g., BVR, MRDD) ❑ _____

Care Planning Decision

Refer to related portions of assessment for review of guidelines that assisted in decision-making.

❑ DO NOT PROCEED—presents little/no risk for problems, has adequate coping skills and/or strategies in place; does not require clinical intervention for:

❑ Cognition ❑ Mood ❑ Behavior ❑ Well Being

❑ PROCEED TO CARE PLANNING FOR **COGNITION**—resident has compromised communication skills creating:

❑ ADL issues ❑ Mood concerns ❑ Well Being issues ❑ Behavior problems ❑ Adjustment problems

❑ Other _____

❑ PROCEED TO CARE PLANNING FOR **MOOD**—resident has:

❑ Adjustment problems ❑ Communication issues ❑ Well Being issues ❑ Behavior problems impacting on mood

❑ Other _____

❑ PROCEED TO CARE PLANNING FOR **BEHAVIOR**—resident has:

❑ Adjustment problems ❑ Cognitive compromise ❑ Well Being issues ❑ Mood problems impacting on Behavior

❑ Other _____

❑ PROCEED TO CARE PLANNING FOR **WELL BEING**—resident has:

❑ Adjustment problems ❑ Cognitive issues ❑ Behavioral problems ❑ Mood problems impacting on Well Being

❑ PROCEED TO CARE PLANNING—*REQUIRES TEACHING* related to _____

Signature/Title of evaluator _____ Date _____

Social Services Quarterly and Periodic Assessment

Name _____ Date of Review _____

Type of Review: ❑ 5-day   ❑ 14-day   ❑ 30-day   ❑ 60-day   ❑ 90-day

Responses should encompass the time frame from last assessment completed. If significant deviation from usual/average occurs within seven days of MDS reference date, clarify in comments section.

I. Cognitive Patterns   Check all that apply.

COGNITIVE STATUS since last assessment: ❑ Unchanged   ❑ Improved   ❑ Deteriorated

Short-Term Memory intact? ❑ Yes ❑ No

Long-Term Memory intact? ❑ Yes ❑ No

Memory/Recall: ❑ Current season   ❑ Location of room   ❑ That in a nursing facility   ❑ Staff names/faces   ❑ None of these

Oriented to: ❑ Time of day   ❑ Day of week   ❑ Month of year   ❑ Year   ❑ None of these

Ability to Think AND Make Decisions: ❑ Decisions consistent and reasonable   ❑ Difficulty making decisions in new situations

❑ Poor decisions, needs cues   ❑ Never/rarely makes decisions   ❑ Easily distracted   ❑ Episodes of disorganized speech

❑ Periods of restlessness   ❑ Periods of lethargy   ❑ Mental status varies   ❑ Different from usual functioning/resident/family or caregivers

Additional remarks, status clarification _____

_____

II. Communication Patterns

COMMUNICATION PATTERNS since last assessment: ❑ Unchanged   ❑ Improved   ❑ Deteriorated

Ability to understand: ❑ Always   ❑ Usually   ❑ Sometimes   ❑ Never/Almost never

Ability to be understood: ❑ Always   ❑ Usually   ❑ Sometimes   ❑ Never/Almost never

Adaptive Equipment Used ❑ Glasses   ❑ Hearing aid   ❑ Communication board   ❑ Other _____

Additional remarks, status clarification _____

_____

III. Mood, Well Being, and Behavior Patterns

MOOD since last assessment: ❑ Unchanged   ❑ Improved   ❑ Deteriorated

Verbal expressions of distress: ❑ Suicidal thoughts   ❑ Negative self statements   ❑ Repetitive questions   ❑ Repetitive verbalization

❑ Persistent anger   ❑ Self deprecation   ❑ Expression of unreal fears   ❑ Statements that something bad about to happen

❑ Repetitive health complaints   ❑ Repetitive complaints/concerns

Sleep Cycle: ❑ Unpleasant mood in morning   ❑ Insomnia/Changes in sleep pattern

Sadness, Apathy, Loss of Interest: ❑ Sad/pained/worried facial expression   ❑ Crying/tearful   ❑ Withdrawn from Activities

❑ Reduced social interaction   ❑ Takes little/no initiative

❑ Mood indicators not present or easily altered

❑ Mood indicators not easily altered

Social Services Quarterly and Periodic Assessment (cont.)

WELL BEING since last assessment: ❏ Unchanged ❏ Improved ❏ Deteriorated

❏ At ease interacting ❏ At ease doing planned activities ❏ Accepts invitations to groups ❏ At ease with self initiated activities

❏ Pursues involvement in NF life ❏ Establishes own goals

_____

_____

BEHAVIOR since last assessment: ❏ Unchanged ❏ Improved ❏ Deteriorated

* Respond on average since last assessment. Use remarks section to clarify any changes in occurrence past seven days.

Wanders: ❏ Never/rarely ❏ 1–3 days/wk ❏ 4–6 days/wk ❏ Daily or more

Verbally Abusive: ❏ Never/rarely ❏ 1–3 days/wk ❏ 4–6 days/wk ❏ Daily or more

Physically Abusive: ❏ Never/rarely ❏ 1–3 days/wk ❏ 4–6 days/wk ❏ Daily or more

Socially Inappropriate /Disruptive: ❏ Never/rarely ❏ 1–3 days/wk ❏ 4–6 days/wk ❏ Daily or more

Resistive to care efforts: ❏ Never/rarely ❏ 1–3 days/wk ❏ 4–6 days/wk ❏ Daily or more

❏ Behaviors not present or easily altered

❏ Behavior present and not easily altered

_____

_____

IV. Physical Restraints and Devices	❏ NA—Skip to next section.

Added since last assessment? ❏ Yes ❏ No **Informed consent in place?** ❏ Yes ❏ No

FUNCTIONAL STATUS since last assessment: ❏ Unchanged ❏ Improved ❏ Deteriorated

Type of device being used: ❏ Side rails ❏ Geri-chair ❏ Jacket ❏ Belt ❏ Recliner ❏ Other

Stated reason for use: ❏ Treat medical symptoms ❏ Behavior management ❏ Supportive device

Does resident want the restraint/device? ❏ No ❏ Yes, reason: _____

Non-medical interventions in place ❏ Yes ❏ No, reason: _____

Further reduction/elimination under way or possible ❏ Yes ❏ No, reason: _____

Remarks _____

_____

_____

_____

_____

Social Services Quarterly and Periodic Assessment (cont.)

V. Psychoactive medication   ❑ NA—Skip to next section.

Added since last assessment? ❑ Yes ❑ No

Mood, Behavior, Well being: ❑ Unchanged   ❑ Improved   ❑ Deteriorated

Type of Drug: ❑ Antipsychotic   ❑ Long-acting anti-anxiety   ❑ Short-acting anti-anxiety   ❑ Antidepressant   ❑ Hypnotic   ❑ Other

Name of drug: _____   **Reason for use:** _____

Non-medical interventions in place? ❑ Yes ❑ No, reason: _____

Further reduction/elimination underway or possible ❑ Yes ❑ No, reason: _____

Remarks _____

_____

VI. Discharge Potential and Overall Status

Advanced Care Directives? ❑ Not desired   ❑ Present, remain applicable   ❑ Present but change

Comments: _____

Indicates preference to return to community? ❑ Yes ❑ No

Support person positive about discharge? ❑ Yes ❑ No

Discharge: ❑ Not anticipated   ❑ Uncertain/unknown   ❑ Within 30 days   ❑ Within 31–90 days

Impact on resident: _____

For additional remarks since last review, add trailer sheet

Social service care planning:

❑ Not indicated   ❑ Remains appropriate   ❑ Will be initiated and/or modified

Signature/Title of evaluator or person completing RAP _____

Dietary Assessment and RAP Review: Nutrition, Hydration, and Tube Feeding

Name _____ DOB _____

Review Date _____ Type of Review: ❑ Adm.   ❑ Annual   ❑ Sig. Change   ❑ Other

Interview Conducted with: ❑ Resident   ❑ Family   ❑ Both   ❑ Significant other   ❑ None of these

Nutritionally Pertinent Diagnosis: _____

I. DIETARY HISTORY/USUAL MEAL PATTERNS—Complete shaded area only at initial admission.

Hx of eating between meals all or most days? ❑ No ❑ Yes   Tobacco products used daily? ❑ No ❑ Yes

Hx use of alcoholic beverages at least weekly? ❑ No ❑ Yes, _____

Distinct food preferences? ❑ No ❑ Yes, _____

Food Allergies? ❑ No ❑ Yes, _____

Portion Size: ❑ Small   ❑ Average   ❑ Large   Usual Amount Eaten: ❑ 25%   ❑ 50%   ❑ 75%   ❑ 100%

Breakfast Time: _____   Typical foods eaten: _____

Lunch Time: _____   Typical foods eaten: _____

Dinner Time: _____   Typical foods eaten: _____

Snacks Time: _____   Typical foods eaten: _____

Nutritional approaches	Type	Additional remarks
❑ Parenteral/IV		
❑ Feeding tube		
❑ Mechanically altered		
❑ Therapeutic diet		
❑ Regular diet		
❑ Syringe fed		
❑ Supplements		
❑ Plate guard, built up utensils, etc.		
❑ Planned weight-change program		

MEDICATIONS: List only those that can alter taste or thirst perception/intake and/or have potential drug/food interactions.

DRUG _____ DOSE _____ EFFECT _____

DRUG _____ DOSE _____ EFFECT _____

Lab test	Date	Result/significance	Test	Date	Result/significance
NA			Total protein		
CL			Albumin		
HGB/HCT			Bun		
RBC			Creatinine		
FE			Glucose		
K+			Cholesterol		
CA			Triglycerides		

Dietary Assessment and RAP Review: Nutrition, Hydration, and Tube Feeding (cont.)

II. WEIGHT HISTORY AND NUTRITIONAL NEEDS

Height: _____ Ft _____ In **Frame Size:** ❑ Small ❑ Medium ❑ Large **Wrist Measurement:** _____

Weight History: Current _____ Usual _____ IBW _____ Adj BW/ % IBW _____

Significant Loss: Last 30 days of 5% ❑ Yes ❑ No Last 180 days of 10%? ❑ Yes ❑ No

Significant Gain: Last 30 days of 5% ❑ Yes ❑ No Last 180 days of 10%? ❑ Yes ❑ No

If weight change, was it unplanned/unexpected? ❑ Yes ❑ No

BEE _____ x Activity Factor _____ x Stress Factor _____ +/- _____ lbs adjusted for weight loss/gain = _____ KCALS

Calculated Protein Needs _____ Calories _____ Fluid _____

III. MENTAL STATUS/BEHAVIOR—Evaluate need/implications of any problems on nutritional status.

Alert, oriented, makes needs known	❑ Yes	❑ No	Paces/wanders	❑ Yes	❑ No
Alertness varies through day	❑ Yes	❑ No	Paranoid/fearful about food/liquid	❑ Yes	❑ No
Anxious behavior affects intake	❑ Yes	❑ No	Sad mood or depression affect intake	❑ Yes	❑ No
Attention span short/easily distracted	❑ Yes	❑ No	Understands/complies with diet	❑ Yes	❑ No
Complains often about food taste	❑ Yes	❑ No	Understands need to eat	❑ Yes	❑ No
Complains regularly/often of hunger	❑ Yes	❑ No	Uses food to gain attention	❑ Yes	❑ No

IV. ORAL/DENTAL CONCERNS—Evaluate need/implications of any problems on nutritional status.

Chewing problems (cavities, broken, missing teeth)	❑ Yes	❑ No	Lips, oral mucosa pale/dry	❑ Yes	❑ No
Dentures present, not used	❑ Yes	❑ No	Mouth pain	❑ Yes	❑ No
Fear of swallowing, choking	❑ Yes	❑ No	Squirrels/cheeks food	❑ Yes	❑ No
Ill fitting/missing dentures	❑ Yes	❑ No	Tongue swollen/coated/inflamed	❑ Yes	❑ No
Inability to swallow	❑ Yes	❑ No	Other _____	❑ Yes	❑ No
Dental referral indicated	❑ Yes	❑ No	Speech therapy recommended	❑ Yes	❑ No

Signature/Title of evaluator or person completing RAP _____

Dietary Assessment and RAP Review: Nutrition, Hydration, and Tube Feeding (cont.)

V. SKIN CONDITION—Evaluate need/implications of any problems on nutritional status.

Pressure Ulcers	❏ Yes	❏ No	Stasis Ulcers	❏ Yes	❏ No	Hx of either	❏ Yes	❏ No
Surgical Wounds	❏ Yes	❏ No	Burns	❏ Yes	❏ No	Healing complications	❏ Yes	❏ No
Poor turgor, thin skin	❏ Yes	❏ No	Dry, flaky	❏ Yes	❏ No	Rashes/lesions	❏ Yes	❏ No
Skin tears or cuts	❏ Yes	❏ No	Other	❏ Yes	❏ No	Irritation/inflammation	❏ Yes	❏ No

Nutrition hydration interventions in place to manage skin problems? ❏ Yes ❏ No

_____

_____

VI. MUSCULAR CONDITIONS—Evaluate need/implications of any problems on nutritional status.

Contractures/paralysis interferes with ability to eat	❏ Yes	❏ No
General weakness/muscle wasting	❏ Yes	❏ No
Poor dexterity/difficulty grasping/holding cup/utensils	❏ Yes	❏ No
Poor balance/inability to sit upright	❏ Yes	❏ No
Twitching/cramping/pain	❏ Yes	❏ No

_____

_____

VII. HEALTH/MEDICAL CONDITIONS—Evaluate need/implications of any problems on nutritional status.

Hx constipation/impaction	❏ Yes	❏ No	Diarrhea	❏ Yes	❏ No	Nausea/Vomiting	❏ Yes	❏ No
Heartburn/indigestion/reflux	❏ Yes	❏ No	Diabetes	❏ Yes	❏ No	CHF/HTN/Arrhythmia	❏ Yes	❏ No
COPD/lung disease/SOB	❏ Yes	❏ No	UTIs	❏ Yes	❏ No	Renal	❏ Yes	❏ No
Radiation therapy	❏ Yes	❏ No	Cancer	❏ Yes	❏ No	Chemotherapy	❏ Yes	❏ No
Dialysis	❏ Yes	❏ No	Liver	❏ Yes	❏ No	Fluid retention/Edema	❏ Yes	❏ No
Fractured bones	❏ Yes	❏ No				Psychoactive drug use	❏ Yes	❏ No

_____

_____

VIII. DEHYDRATION RISK FACTORS—Evaluate need/implications of any problems on nutritional status.

Decreased thirst perception	❏ Yes	❏ No	Restricted fluids due to health reasons	❏ Yes	❏ No
Excessive sweating/fever/infection	❏ Yes	❏ No	Restricts fluid intake to avoid incontinence	❏ Yes	❏ No
Mucous membranes dry	❏ Yes	❏ No	Uses laxatives/enemas/diuretics	❏ Yes	❏ No
Poor intake by history	❏ Yes	❏ No	Urine output exceeds 2000cc/day	❏ Yes	❏ No
Refuses/unaware of need for fluids	❏ Yes	❏ No	Urine volume concentrated	❏ Yes	❏ No

_____

_____

Signature/Title of evaluator or person completing RAP _____

Dietary Assessment and RAP Review: Nutrition, Hydration, and Tube Feeding (cont.)

IX. TUBE FEEDING ASSESSMENT   ❑ NA—Skip section

Initial Placement Date _____ Type of Tube _____

Reason for Placement _____ Expected Removal Date _____

Alternatives tried? ❑ Yes ❑ No, reason: _____

Product _____ Amount _____ Route _____

Rate _____ Other liquids provided _____

TF/ Fluids Provided _____ KCALS _____ Protein _____

Fluids _____ Free H₂0 _____ RDAs _____

Calculate total for all parenteral/IV received since MDS assessment reference date					

PORTION OF TOTAL DAILY CALORIES: ❑ None   ❑ 1–25%   ❑ 26–50%   ❑ 51–75%   ❑ 76–100%

PORTION OF DAILY FLUID INTAKE: ❑ NA   ❑ 1–500 cc   ❑ 501–1000 cc   ❑ 1001–1500 cc   ❑ 1501–2000 cc   ❑ 2001 cc +

Complicating Factors and Risk Occurrence

❑ Abdominal distension/pain	❑ Agitation	❑ Constipation	❑ Epistaxis	❑ Pneumonia
❑ Airway obstruction	❑ Depression	❑ Fecal impaction	❑ Respiratory distress	❑ Dehydration
❑ Limb restraints	❑ Self extubation	❑ Anxiety	❑ Diarrhea	❑ Obesity
❑ Aspiration	❑ Displacement of tube	❑ Other _____		

Recommendations/remarks. (Indicate if alternatives and/or weaning is possible. Note any adjustments needed to tube feeding based on calculations and presence of risk factors.)

_____

_____

IX. CARE PLANNING DECISIONS

❑ **DO NOT PROCEED** TO CARE PLANNING NUTRITION—Little to no risk for compromise is present.

❑ **PROCEED** TO NUTRITIONAL CARE PLANNING—Compromised status, risk factors, and/or complications indicate need for intervention. Refer to information and evaluation of guidelines contained throughout this assessment.

❑ **DO NOT PROCEED** TO CARE PLANNING DEHYDRATION—Little to no risk is present as indicated in section VIII.

❑ **PROCEED** TO CARE PLANNING FOR DEHYDRATION for factors noted in section VIII.

❑ **PROCEED** TO CARE PLANNING TUBE FEEDING, related to factors noted under section IX.

❑ **PROCEED** TO CARE PLANNING—REQUIRES TEACHING related to _____

_____

_____

_____

_____

Dietary Quarterly and Periodic Assessment

Resident Name _____ Date _____

Type of Review: ❑ 5-day ❑ 14-day ❑ 30-day ❑ 60-day ❑ 90-day ❑ Other

Responses should encompass the time frame from last assessment completed. If significant deviation from usual/average occurs within seven days of MDS reference date clarify in comments section.

ORAL/NUTRITIONAL STATUS

Oral Problems: ❑ Chewing problems ❑ Swallowing problems ❑ Mouth pain

Weight Changes: ❑ No ❑ Loss 5% last 30 days ❑ Gain 5% last 30 days ❑ Loss 10% last 180 days ❑ Gain 10% last 180 days

Nutritional Problems: ❑ C/O taste of many foods ❑ Regular C/O of hunger ❑ Leaves 25% or more uneaten most meals

Eating Assistance: ❑ Independent ❑ Supervised ❑ Limited assist ❑ Extensive assist ❑ Total dependence

_____

_____

APPROACHES

❑ Mech altered _____ ❑ Therapeutic diet _____ ❑ Supplements _____

❑ Adaptive device _____ ❑ Planned wt change program _____

❑ Nutrition/hydration interventions to manage skin problems ❑ Syringe fed ❑ Parenteral/IV feeding _____

FOR PARENTERAL/ENTERAL ONLY

Calculate total for all parenteral/IV received since MDS assessment reference date.

Portion of total daily calories: ❑ None ❑ 1–25% ❑ 26–50% ❑ 51–75% ❑ 76–100%

Portion of daily fluid intake: ❑ NA ❑ 1-500 cc ❑ 501-1000 cc ❑ 1001-1500 cc ❑ 1501-2000 cc ❑ 2001 cc >

Product _____ Amount _____ Route _____ Rate _____ Other liquids _____

TF/ Fluids Provide _____ KCALS _____ Protein _____ Fluids _____ Free H_2O _____ RDAs _____

SKIN: ❑ Intact ❑ New pressure ulcers since last review ❑ Healing pressure ulcers ❑ Other problems

_____

LABS: ❑ None since last review ❑ WNL or not impacting nutritional status ❑ Abnormal, with nutritional significance, explain: _____

_____

Medication changes, or additions actually or potentially affecting nutrition or hydration.

❑ No ❑ Yes ❑ Possibly ❑ Constipation ❑ Diarrhea ❑ Drowsy at meals ❑ Anorexia ❑ N&V ❑ Altered taste/labs ❑ Tremors ❑ GI distress

❑ Weight gain _____ lbs. ❑ Weight loss _____ lbs. ❑ Other _____

COGNITIVE FUNCTION IMPACTING ON NUTRITION: ❑ NA ❑ No change ❑ Improved ❑ Deteriorated

PSYCHOSOCIAL FUNCTION IMPACTING ON NUTRITION: ❑ NA ❑ No change ❑ Improved ❑ Deteriorated

ADL FUNCTION IMPACTING ON NUTRITION: ❑ NA ❑ No change ❑ Improved ❑ Deteriorated

Explain improvements, declines, or failures to improve when status indicates potential exits. _____

_____

NUTRITIONAL CARE PLANNING ❑ Not indicated ❑ Remains appropriate ❑ Will be initiated and/or modified

Signature/Title of evaluator _____

Nursing Assessment and History

❑ Admission   ❑ Annual

Resident Name _____ Adm. Date _____ Readm. Date _____

Reason for admission: ❑ LT Placement   ❑ Rehab/Recuperation   ❑ Hospice Care   ❑ Respite Care   ❑ Other _____
Admitted From: ❑ Hospital   ❑ Private Home   ❑ Assisted Living   ❑ Retirement Community   ❑ Group Home   ❑ Other _____
Admitting Diagnosis _____
Other Active Diagnosis, Health Conditions _____
Refer to physician order sheet for medications, allergies, and treatments.

Mental Status Assessment   ❑ Comatose (if present skip to section on Physical Assessment Status)
Directions: Check all that apply.

Memory: ❑ Short-term intact   ❑ Not intact, can't remember 3 items in 5 minutes   ❑ Can follow directions
        ❑ Long-term memory intact, knows family and significant life events   ❑ Not intact
Recall: ❑ Knows name   ❑ Current season   ❑ Why s/he was admitted   ❑ No recall
Decision-Making: ❑ Reasonable   ❑ Some difficulty   ❑ Poor   ❑ Rarely/never makes any
Comments, clarification _____
_____

Indicators of Delirium/Disordered Thinking
Directions: If anything other than None is checked, further evaluation is indicated. Alert RN Assessment Coordinator.

❑ None   ❑ Easily distracted   ❑ Thinks s/he elsewhere/confuses day and night   ❑ Speech disorganized   ❑ Restless, fidgets, calling out
❑ Lethargic, difficult to arouse, staring in space   ❑ Mental status varies
Comments, clarification _____

Sensory and Communication (Analysis can eliminate need to complete Vision and Communication RAPs if triggered on MDS)
Directions: Check all that apply. Checks in bolded areas indicated the need for additional action/care planning, proceed accordingly. Non-bolded areas may be considered strengths when addressing other problems/needs on the care plan.

VISION
Eyes: ❑ Clear   ❑ Drainage   ❑ Irritation   ❑ Redness   ❑ Visual, perceptual defect
Pupils: ❑ Equal/reactive   ❑ No, _____
Vision: ❑ Adequate   Inadequate: ❑ Sees only object's outline   ❑ Follows with eyes   ❑ Doesn't follow with eyes   ❑ Blind
❑ Side Vision Compromised: ❑ Left   ❑ Right   ❑ Sees halos, rings, flashes of light   ❑ Eye pain, blurred or double vision
Eye exam: ❑ Done in past 12 months   ❑ Longer   ❑ No or unknown   ❑ Candidate for eye exam
Appliance: ❑ Glasses   ❑ Magnifying glass   ❑ Contacts   ❑ Other
Eye Med: ❑ No   ❑ If yes, received as prescribed ❑ No ❑ Yes
Use is independent? ❑ Yes ❑ No   **Appliance in good repair?** ❑ Yes ❑ No
Functional Impact of vision: ❑ None   ❑ Interferes with ADLs   ❑ Interferes with independence/being involved
Comments, clarification _____

Nursing Assessment and History (cont.)

COMMUNICATION

Ears: ❑ Clean, without wax buildup ❑ Wax impacted ❑ Drainage ❑ Recent change in hearing

Hearing: ❑ Adequate in quiet setting ❑ Impaired: speaker must adjust voice tone/rate/pitch ❑ No useful hearing

Hearing aid: ❑ No ❑ Present: ❑ Used ❑ Doesn't use ❑ Candidate for hearing exam

Speech: ❑ Clear and audible ❑ Inaudible ❑ Unclear, slurred, garbles or nonsensical ❑ Absent

Modes of Expression: ❑ Verbal ❑ Written ❑ Signs/gestures/sounds ❑ Sign language/Braille ❑ Communication board ❑ None ❑ Candidate for speech evaluation

Understands: ❑ Always ❑ Usually ❑ Sometimes ❑ Rarely/Never

Understood: ❑ Always ❑ Usually ❑ Sometimes ❑ Rarely/Never

Comments, clarification _____

_____

Psychosocial Status—Any checks indicating a problem require initial care planning and should also be referred to Social Services for further evaluation.

Well Being: ❑ Accepting of placement ❑ Comfortable, at ease ❑ Distressed over placement ❑ Ill at ease

Expresses feelings: ❑ Readily ❑ With difficulty ❑ Not at all

Problems with relationships: ❑ No ❑ Yes _____

Mood: ❑ Pleasant, Cheerful ❑ Unpleasant, Irritable ❑ Change in sleep cycle ❑ Presents as sad or distressed ❑ Crying, tearful ❑ Repetitive remarks about health concern ❑ Repetitive questions ❑ Negative comments ❑ Fearful ❑ Sense of impending doom ❑ Lacks initiative ❑ Restlessness, paces, fidgets ❑ Withdrawn

Behavior: ❑ Aggressive ❑ Inappropriate actions ❑ Wanders ❑ Verbally or physically abusive ❑ Resistant to care ❑ Restraints are/have been in use to manage behavior ❑ Psychotherapeutic meds are in use or have been used in last 30 days

Comments, clarification _____

_____

Physical Status Assessment

CARDIOPULMONARY

Apical rate: _____ **Radial rate:** _____ **Rhythm:** ❑ Regular ❑ Irregular ❑ Bounding ❑ Thready

Peripheral Pulses Present: ❑ Right ___ Strong ___ Weak ❑ Left ___ Strong ___ Weak ❑ Not present

BP Right Arm: Sitting _____ Standing _____ Lying _____ **Temperature:** _____

BP Left Arm: Sitting _____ Standing _____ Lying _____

Edema: ❑ No ❑ Pitting ❑ Non-pitting Location _____

Complaints of Chest Pain: ❑ No ❑ Yes ___ Constant ___ Intermittent ___ At rest with activity ___ Anxious

Complaints of palpitations or heart racing: ❑ No ❑ Yes ___ Constant ___ Intermittent

Comments, clarification _____

_____

Respiratory Rate: _____ ❑ Unlabored ❑ Labored

Breath sounds: ❑ Clear ❑ Diminished ❑ Congested ❑ Short of breath: ___ Always ___ With exertion ___ At night

Cough: ❑ No ❑ Non-productive ❑ Productive Sputum: ___ yellow ___ green ___ white ___ clear

Treatments: ❑ Suctioning ❑ Trach Care ❑ Oxygen: ___ Continuous ___ PRN ___ Mask ___ Cannula ___ Vent Care

Comments, clarification _____

_____

Signature/Title _____ **Date** _____

 The Big Book of Care Plans, Second Edition

Nursing Assessment and History (cont.)

Elimination
Directions: Check all that apply. If incontinence is present or catheters used alert RN Assessment Coordinator.

BOWEL continence: ❑ Always or **Incontinent**   ❑ Less than weekly   ❑ Weekly 2–3x/wk   ❑ All or most of time

BM Control via: ❑ Ostomy   ❑ Enemas/irrigations   ❑ Scheduled toileting times   ❑ Use of laxatives   ❑ None of these

Habits/Problems: ❑ BM daily or twice weekly   ❑ Constipated, over 3 days between BM   ❑ Diarrhea   ❑ Fecal Impaction

---

BLADDER continence: ❑ Always or **Incontinent**   ❑ Once/week   ❑ Daily   ❑ Always inadequate control

Control of incontinence via: ❑ Catheter   ❑ Scheduled toileting times   ❑ Pads/briefs   ❑ None of these

History: ❑ Able to recognize urges   ❑ Can respond to urges ___ indep. ___ with assist ___ Unable to recognize urges

❑ Spurts urine with coughing/laughing/straining   ❑ Loses large amount of urine on standing/shifting to upright position

❑ Complains of frequency/urgency   ❑ Takes diuretic   ❑ UTI last 30 days   ❑ UTI several times/year

Catheter Use: ❑ Constant   ❑ Intermittent   Reason for Use: _____

Nutrition and Hydration—Any checks indicating a problem require care planning and should also be referred to Dietary.

Height: _____ Ft _____ In   **Weight** _____ lbs.   ❑ Stable   ❑ Unstable

Appears to be: ❑ Above Average wt.   ❑ Average wt.   ❑ Below average wt.

This is: ❑ Usual   ❑ Unusual

Diet: ❑ Regular   ❑ Mechanically Altered   ❑ Therapeutic   ❑ Enteral/Parenteral

Food/Fluid Intake: ❑ By Mouth   ❑ Feeding Tube   ❑ Syringe   ❑ NPO

Level of Assistance: ❑ Independent   ❑ Supervised   ❑ Assisted   ❑ Dependent

Quantity of Food Portions: ❑ Large   ❑ Average   ❑ Small   ❑ Unknown/NA

Appetite: ❑ Good   ❑ Fair   ❑ Poor/None   ❑ Complains of food tastes   ❑ Complains of hunger often

Liquid Intake: ❑ Drinks between meals   ❑ Drinks with meals   ❑ Rarely/Never feels thirsty   ❑ Excessive sweating or fever

Problems: ❑ Chewing   ❑ Swallowing   ❑ Pain in mouth/throat   ❑ Fear of swallowing, choking   ❑ Vomiting, diarrhea, nausea

❑ Anemic, pale mucous membranes   ❑ Abdominal distention present

---

Oral Dental Status (Analysis of this section can eliminate need to complete related RAP if it triggers on MDS.)
Checks in bolded areas may indicate the need for additional action/care planning. Proceed accordingly. Non-bolded areas may be considered strengths when addressing other problems/needs on the care plan.

Condition: ❑ Gums pink, moist   ❑ Coated, bleeding or swollen   ❑ Ulcerated/inflamed   ❑ Mouth pain/sensitivity   ❑ White patches

❑ Mouth odor present   ❑ Tongue/lips/mucosa dry, cracked, or coated

Teeth: ❑ All present   ❑ Some missing   ❑ All missing   ❑ Broken, loose or carious

Dentures: ❑ None   ❑ Full   ❑ Partial   ❑ Bridge   ❑ Does not/cannot wear, reason _____

Oral Care: ❑ Completed on own   ❑ With assist   ❑ Does not/cannot do   ❑ Resists oral care

Other factors: ❑ Has had Rheumatic fever, hip replacement, or has Diabetes or takes anticoagulants   ❑ Embarrassed by condition of teeth

❑ Has not been seen by dentist in past year or since problems have developed

---

Nursing Assessment and History (cont.)

PAIN

Presence: ❑ None ❑ Mild ❑ Moderate ❑ Excruciating ❑ Unable to be determined/seems in distress of some sort

Frequency: ❑ No pain ❑ Less than daily ❑ Daily or more often

Site: ❑ Back ❑ Bone ❑ Chest ❑ Hip ❑ Joint ❑ Stomach ❑ Headache ❑ Incisional ❑ Other _____

Relief from: ❑ Non-medical interventions ❑ Medication ❑ Other _____ ❑ No relief

_____

_____

Skin Condition—Check all that apply and complete risk assessment tool to determine care planning need.

Color: ❑ Pink ❑ Pale ❑ Cyanotic ❑ Jaundiced

Condition: ❑ Dry, flaky ❑ Clammy ❑ Warm ❑ Cold ❑ Poor turgor ❑ Desensitized to pain ❑ Abrasions ❑ Bruises ❑ Burns ❑ Skin tears, cuts ❑ Rash ❑ Surgical wound ❑ Stasis ulcer ❑ Pressure ulcer or history of _____ Foot infection _____ Open lesions, foot _____Corns, calluses, hammer toes, bunions, toes cross, pain

FRONT	BACK	Type of Problem	Location	Stage	Description

Hygiene and Grooming

Bolded areas indicate need for further assessment. Alert RN Assessment Coordinator or Restorative Nurse.

Bathing: ❑ Independent ❑ Supervise ❑ Assist ❑ Dependent ❑ Prompts, direction, task segmentation

Dressing: ❑ Independent ❑ Supervise ❑ Assist ❑ Dependent ❑ Prompts, direction ❑ Street clothes ❑ Bed clothes during day

Hygiene: ❑ Indep. ❑ Supervise ❑ Assist ❑ Dependent ❑ Prompts, direction

Preferences: ❑ Tub ❑ Shower ❑ Bed bath ❑ Female assist ❑ Male assist ❑ AM ❑ PM

_____

_____

Mobility

Also do fall-risk assessment. Bolded areas reflect need for further assessment. Alert RN Assessment Coordinator or Restorative Nurse.

Ambulation: ❑ Indep. ❑ Supervise ❑ Assist ❑ Dependent ❑ Prompts, direction

Transfer: ❑ Indep. ❑ Supervise ❑ Assist ❑ Dependent ❑ Prompts, direction, balance

Gait: ❑ Unsteady ❑ Needs support to sit upright ❑ Needs support to stand/walk

Disabilities: ❑ Paraplegic ❑ Quadriplegic ❑ Hemiplegia: L R ❑ Poor coordination, dexterity problem

Limited Range of Motion: ❑ Neck ❑ Arm: L R ❑ Hand: L R ❑ Leg: L R ❑ Foot: L R ❑ Other

Appliance/Equipment: ❑ Wheelchair ❑ Walker ❑ Cane ❑ Splint/Brace ❑ Use of restraint for support*

_____

_____

Nursing Assessment and History (cont.)

Side Rail Safety Assessment
Evaluate if side rails are or are not indicated. Obtain order if use indicated.

Side Rail Use is: ❑ Not indicated   ❑ Indicated: ❑ Full or 3/4   ❑ Half   ❑ One side   ❑ Both Sides
❑ Permits getting in/out of bed unassisted   ❑ Allows increased mobility
❑ Resident demands use, reason: _____   ❑ Resident refuses use, reason: _____
❑ Use provides safety due to physical size and dependence when turning   ❑ Active seizure disorder
❑ Use prompts to request assist   ❑ Use needed to prevent getting out of bed
(THIS IS A RESTRAINT AND DEMANDS EXPANDED ASSESSMENT)

Safety Risk with Use: ❑ Going over rail/out end of bed/falls   ❑ Skin tears   ❑ Bruises   ❑ Abrasions   ❑ Entrapment   ❑ Other

Safety Risk without Use: ❑ Falling out of bed   ❑ Falling while self transferring   ❑ Difficulty mobilizing   ❑ Anxiety   ❑ Other

_____

_____

Signature/Title _____ Date _____

Psychotropic Drug Side Effect Monitor

Antipsychotic, Antidepressants, Anti-Anxiety, Hypnotics

Resident Name _____

Drug Name	Frequency	Reason for use
_____	_____	_____
_____	_____	_____
_____	_____	_____

ADDRESS ALL THAT APPLY	Date		Date		Date		Date		Date		Date		Date	
	Y	N	Y	N	Y	N	Y	N	Y	N	Y	N	Y	N
Depression present or worsened														
Decline in Mood/Behavior ADL														
Hallucinations/delusions present or worsened														
Cognition worse or recently impaired														
Acute confusion not r/t to severe depression/medical illness														
Sedation or drowsiness since med(s)														
Slurred speech														
Gait/balance disturbance														
Urinary incontinence worsened or recently developed														
Falls														
Dry mouth														
General status decline since med(s)														
INITIALS OF REVIEWER														

Complete only when using Antipsychotic Medication.

If Y response, complete more definitive test such as AIMS.

	Y	N	Y	N	Y	N	Y	N	Y	N	Y	N	Y	N
Orthostatic Hypotension Systolic drop 20 pts sit to stand or C/o dizziness, loss of balance from lying to sit/stand position														
Tremors, unsteadiness, pill rolling. Rigidity of limb, neck, trunk, or shuffling gait														
Akinesia: Marked decrease in spontaneous movement														
Dystonia: Holds self in rigid unnatural position														
Akathisia: Unable to sit still														
Tardive Dyskinesia: involuntary movements (e.g., thrusting, chewing movements)														
Parkinson's disease														
INITIALS OF REVIEWER														

Signature/Title of evaluator or person completing RAP _____

Psychoactive Drug Use Progress Note

Indicate presence or absence of side effects and any change in side effects since last assessment. Indicate the impact of medication on mood and behavior.

Resident Name _____ Date _____

_____
_____
_____
_____

Team Member(s) Completing _____ Date _____

_____
_____
_____
_____

Team Member(s) Completing _____ Date _____

_____
_____
_____
_____

Team Member(s) Completing _____ Date _____

_____
_____
_____
_____

Team Member(s) Completing _____

Signature/Title of evaluator or person completing RAP _____

Side Rail Safety Assessment

Resident Name _____

Directions: Think **Safety First** when considering using or not using a side rail; is the resident at risk? Remember, totally independent and totally immobile residents generally present little risk. Consider the level of capability and disability in your decision-making process. Consider the following, then complete the appropriate section.

Bed mobility:	Level of independence/ability to move about; need for and degree of assistance.
Transfer capacity:	Level of independence/supervision needed; attempt or lack of attempt to transfer with or without assistance.
Capacity to ambulate:	Need/level of assistance to walk, hands on or mechanical; need/level of assistance if chair-/bedfast.
Toileting:	Continence status, ability to recognize/respond to urges.
Cognitive status:	Awareness of limitations, safety factors, comprehension, retention.
Sleep/wake cycles:	Presence of pain.

SIDE RAILS ARE NOT INDICATED

Reason for Non-Use: ❏ Totally independent ❏ Totally immobile ❏ Promote independence
❏ Minimize injury caused by attempts to get out of bed unassisted ❏ Other _____

Potential Risk: ❏ None ❏ Yes, specify _____

Interventions to Minimize Risk: ❏ N/A ❏ Lock bed castors/ensure furniture secure ❏ Lower bed height ❏ Use fall mat
❏ Non-slip carpet ❏ Anticipate needs (refer to care plan) ❏ Other _____

SIDE RAILS ARE INDICATED: ❏ Full ❏ Half ❏ One side ❏ Both sides

Reason for Use: ❏ To prevent getting out of bed (This is a restraint and requires expanded assessment) ❏ Allow increased bed mobility
❏ Safety due to physical size ❏ Seizure disorder ❏ Safety due to visual/special deficits ❏ Dependence in turning
❏ Totally dependent in mobility ❏ Prompt to request assist ❏ Other _____

Safety Risk with Use: ❏ None ❏ Going over rail/out end of bed/falls ❏ Skin tears ❏ Bruises ❏ Abrasions
❏ Entrapment ❏ Other _____

Risk if Not Used: ❏ Falling out of bed ❏ Reduced bed mobility ❏ Anxiety/Fear ❏ Other _____

Interventions to Minimize Risk: ❏ N/A ❏ Pad rails ❏ Eliminate gaps between mattress/end of bed
❏ Call light kept within reach ❏ Anticipate needs (toileting, thirst, hunger, boredom)
❏ Other _____

Resident/Family in agreement with side rail decisions and understands benefit risk.
❏ Yes ❏ No, reason: _____

Comments/clarification _____
_____

Signature/Title of evaluator or person completing RAP _____

Status Evaluation for Use of Physical Restraints

Resident Name _____

Type of Restraint	Reason for Use	Duration of Application

Directions: Complete on initiation of restraint use, four times weekly, then monthly. Use progress notes on reverse side to explain any changes from one assessment to the next. Aggressive action is indicated if symptoms develop. If they are not related to use of restraint there must clear documentation as to why not.

Symptoms	Date		Date		Date		Date		Date		Date		Date	
	Y	N	Y	N	Y	N	Y	N	Y	N	Y	N	Y	N
Cognitive skills worsened														
Depression present or worse														
Hallucination/delusions present/worse														
Withdrawn/decline in initiative														
Seems sleepy/sleeping much of day														
Decline in behavior/mood/well being														
Decline in ADL/increased dependence														
Decline in mobility/increase in dependence														
Decline in sitting/standing balance														
Decline in range of motion														
Urinary incontinence present/worse														
Constipation present/worse														
Weight loss/loss of appetite														
Symptoms of dehydration														
Pressure sore(s)														
Infection														
Falls														
INITIALS														

Signature/Title of evaluator or person completing RAP _____

Physical Restraint Use Progress Note

Indicate the impact of the restraint use on the resident. Clarify changes from one assessment to the next. Indicate actions initiated if new side effects are noted.

Resident Name _____ Date _____

_____

_____

_____

_____

Team Member(s) Completing _____ Date _____

_____

_____

_____

_____

Team Member(s) Completing _____ Date _____

_____

_____

_____

_____

Team Member(s) Completing _____ Date _____

_____

_____

_____

_____

Team Member(s) Completing _____

Signature/Title of evaluator or person completing RAP _____

Nurse's Notes: Skin Integrity

Directions: Note skin-risk assessment scores as they are done. Read each statement, checking response as appropriate. Explain any no response in adjacent nurse's notes. In general, any reddened area will require a review of the care plan.

DATE		Yes	No	Yes	No	Yes	No	Yes	No	Yes	No	Yes	No	Yes	No
RISK SCORE															
Skin intact															
Without reddened area(s)															
If pressure ulcer, skin grid reflects stable/improving															
Consumes 75% to 100% most meals															
Supplements are provided															
Supplements consumed most of time															
Fluid intake/hydration status is adequate															
Drinks most fluids offered and provided															
Skin protocol is consistently followed															
Cooperative with care															
Care Plan effective, continue interventions															
Nurse's Initials															

Structured Nurse's Note: Continence Management Programs

Resident Name	Program Initiation Date

Type of Program: ❑ Habit training ❑ Schedules Toileting ❑ Prompted Voiding ❑ Check and Change

Date	Yes	No	Yes	No	Yes	No	Yes	No	Yes	No	Yes	No	Yes	No
Interventions are initiated within 15 minutes of scheduled time.														
Resident is cooperative with EACH toileting/care intervention.														
Resident responds to interventions needed for toileting activities.														
Skin is intact, without rash, etc, in perinea/buttocks area.														
Clothes and undergarments are kept dry and odor free.														
Established goals are in process of being met and/or have been met and are stable.														
Nurse's Initials Shift _____														

Directions: Check yes or no for each statement. Explain any NO responses using nurse's notes beginning on reverse side. Complete on initiation of program daily, each shift used, x 7 days, then weekly x 3, then monthly x 2. Once program is firmly established (approximately 3 months), eliminate this tool and use Comprehensible Nurse's Note format to reflect service delivery and status.

Nurse's Notes

Directions: Read each statement, checking response as appropriate. Explain any NO response in narrative nurse's notes on reverse side.

DATE															
	Yes	No	Yes	No	Yes	No	Yes	No	Yes	No	Yes	No	Yes	No
Nurse's Initials															

© 2009 HCPro, Inc.

Seven-Day Core ADL Tracking Tool

Resident Name _____ Start Date _____ End Date _____

DIRECTIONS: Review each activity and note the **GREATEST NUMBER of times** (up to 3) that help was provided of any kind in each category. Also reflect at the bottom of each column the **GREATEST AMOUNT** of support provided: 1 person or 2 person assist.

SHIFT _____		Bed Mobility							Eating							Transfer							Toileting						
HELP PROVIDED	Day	1	2	3	4	5	6	7	1	2	3	4	5	6	7	1	2	3	4	5	6	7	1	2	3	4	5	6	7
Independent *Place a check mark ONLY IF:* Resident did TOTALLY ON OWN																													
Total Care *Place a check mark ONLY IF:* Resident did ABSOLUTELY NOTHING FOR SELF; STAFF DID EVERYTHING																													
Supervised Resident completed the activity BUT REQUIRED CLUES, SUPERVISION, OVERSIGHT TO DO THE TASK																													
Limited Assistance Resident very involved in helping self BUT STAFF ASSISTED/GUIDED ACTIVITY																													
Extensive Assistance Resident helped very little AND STAFF PROVIDED WEIGHT-BEARING ASSISTANCE (CARRIED *ANY* PART OF RESIDENT WEIGHT)																													
Total number of staff helping with activity																													
Initials of person completing the information																													

Seven-Day Mood and Behavior Tracker

Name _____ START DATE _____

Directions: Check all that apply each day.

BE SURE YOU REVIEW <u>EACH</u> ITEM <u>EACH</u> DAY. THIS INFORMATION MUST BE ACCURATE!

DAY SHIFT	1	2	3	4	5	6	7
Made negative statements							
Repetitive questions, repetitive calling out for help							
Angry at self or others, runs self down							
Unrealistic fears and/or feels something bad is about to happen							
Complains about health							
Anxious complaints/concerns other than health							
Unpleasant mood on waking							
Sad, pained, worried facial expressions; crying, tearful							
Repetitive physical movements (e.g., pacing, hand wringing, etc.)							
Withdrawn, disinterested in surroundings							
CHEERS UP EASILY (Y = Yes, N = No)							
Wanders without purpose							
Screams, threatens, curses							
Hits, shoves, scratches, attempts to sexually abuse others							
Socially inappropriate or disruptive behavior							
Resists care							
BEHAVIOR EASILY ALTERED (Y = Yes, N = No)							
Complains of pain or appears to be in pain							
Slept or dozed longer than 1 hour this shift							
Spends time in leisure activities, pursues own interest							
YOUR INITIALS							

EVENING SHIFT	1	2	3	4	5	6	7
Made negative statements							
Repetitive questions, repetitive calling out for help							
Angry at self or others, runs self down							
Unrealistic fears and/or feels something bad is about to happen							
Complains about health, anxious, complaints/concerns other than health							
Sad, pained, worried facial expressions; crying, tearful							
Repetitive physical movements (e.g., pacing, hand wringing, etc.)							
Withdrawn, disinterested in surroundings							
CHEERS UP EASILY (Y = Yes, N = No)							
Wanders without purpose							
Screams, threatens, curses							
Hits, shoves, scratches, attempts to sexually abuse others							
Socially inappropriate or disruptive behavior							
Resists care							
BEHAVIOR EASILY ALTERED (Y = Yes, N = No)							
Complains of pain or appears to be in pain							
Slept or dozed longer than 1 hour prior to retiring for night							
Spends time in leisure activities, pursues own interest							
YOUR INITIALS							

Seven-Day Mood and Behavior Tracker (cont.)

NIGHT SHIFT	1	2	3	4	5	6	7
Complains of pain or appears to be in pain							
Verbally abusive							
Physically abusive							
Wanders without purpose							
Socially inappropriate							
Resists care							
Problems sleeping, up more than once							
Sad, anxious, depressed							
Spends time in leisure activities (e.g., reading, radio, tv)							
BEHAVIOR EASILY ALTERED, EASILY CHEERED UP (Y= Yes N= No)							
YOUR INITIALS							

Completing the ADL TRACKER

1. Insert the following codes at the end of each shift.

2. For best results, have the licensed nurse obtain the information from the direct-care staff at the end of each shift.

Column R: Code what the RESIDENT DID FOR SELF

0 = Independent

1 = Cues, oversight, encouragement (supervision)

2 = Very involved in the activity (limited assist)

3 = Resident helped minimally (extensive assist)

4 = Did not participate in any way (total care)

Column S: Code the MOST help given

0 = No help needed/given

1 = set-up help provided

2 = 1 person helped

3 = 2 + people helped

N/A = Not applicable

ADL Directives

Resident Name _____ Date Initiated _____

> **Purpose:** To provide direct-care staff with individualized information to meet the day-to-day care needs of the resident.
>
> **Direction:** Check all that apply; use MDS to assist. List interventions staff is to use in meeting day-to-day care needs.

MENTAL STATUS AND DECISION-MAKING

❏ Recalls day to day   ❏ Recalls past life experiences   ❏ Status varies throughout day   ❏ Knows season

❏ Knows location of room   ❏ Recognizes staff names/faces   ❏ Never makes decisions   ❏ None of these

❏ Decisions consistent/reasonable   ❏ Poor (i.e.) _____

COMMUNICATION, HEARING, VISION

Understands:	❏ Always	❏ Usually	❏ Sometimes	❏ Never
Understood:	❏ Always	❏ Usually	❏ Occasionally	❏ Never
Speech:	❏ No speech	❏ Clear	❏ Unclear (i.e.) _____	
Hearing:	❏ No problem	❏ Some difficulty	❏ Absence useful hearing	
Hearing aid:	❏ No	❏ Yes Left Right		
Vision:	❏ Able to see	❏ Wears glasses	❏ Needs to put on/take off ❏ Not able to see ❏ Artificial eye L R	

Interventions needed _____

_____

MOOD AND BEHAVIOR

❏ Mood generally good   ❏ Mood is often sad/unhappy (i.e.) _____

❏ Behavior generally reasonable   ❏ Behavior is often problematic (i.e.) _____

Suggested manner of approach _____

_____

SPECIAL CONSIDERATIONS

Prefers to be called _____

Needs/wants from staff (Note particular preferences or things that make resident feel better, s/he enjoys talking about, etc.)

> ❏ **Fall-Risk Precautions:** ❏ Bed alarm   ❏ Chair alarm   ❏ Other _____
>
> ❏ **Skin-Risk Precautions:** _____
>
> ❏ **PHYSICAL RESTRAINT:** ❏ Belt   ❏ Jacket   ❏ G/C   ❏ Lap buddy   ❏ Wrist   ❏ Mitt   ❏ Merry walker   ❏ Side rails
>
> ❏ Other _____
>
> Time period for use: _____
>
> Circumstances of use: _____
>
> YOU MUST CHECK EVERY 15-30 MINUTES AND EXERCISE EVERY 1–2 HOURS PER POC

ADL Directives (cont.)

Resident Self Performance Code based on AVERAGE performance   NA = Not applicable/not done

I = Independent, no help or occasional support   **S** = Supervision, oversight, encouragement, cueing

LA = Limited assist, resident very involved   **EA** = Extensive assist, resident does some, staff does most   **T** = Does nothing for Self

Staff Support Codes   Code based on AVERAGE support   NA = Not applicable/not done

0 = No setup or physical help   **1** = Setup help only   **2** = One person physical assist   **3** = Two + person physical assist

Resident Performance	Staff Support	Special Instructions, Task Segmentation Needed, Comments, Clarifications Indicate type of supervision and what type of assist needed if LA or EA.
Bed Mobility ❑ Side rails for mobility		**Restorative Nursing Program** ❑ No ❑ Yes _____ **APPLIANCES/DEVICES:** ❑ Ted Hose ❑ Splint Brace _____ ❑ Other _____
Transfer ❑ Bedfast ❑ Lifted ❑ Hoyer ❑ Side rails for transfer		
Walking in Room		
Walking in Hall		
Locomotion on Unit ❑ Cane/Walker ❑ W/C ❑ G/C		
Eating ❑ NPO ❑ NG ❑ G-tube ❑ Other _____		**Restorative Dining Program** ❑ Yes ❑ No **Adaptive Equipment** ❑ Yes ❑ No **Diet** _____ **Supplements** _____
Toilet Use **Continent Bladder** ❑ Yes ❑ No **Catheter** ❑ External ❑ Internal **Continent Bowel** ❑ Yes ❑ No ❑ Colostomy		❑ **Continence Management Program** **Uses** ❑ bathroom ❑ bedside ❑ commode ❑ urinal ❑ bedpan **Toilet schedule** _____ ❑ 1st shift ❑ 2nd shift ❑ 3rd shift **Adult pads** ❑ N/A ❑ Always ❑ Day ❑ Night ❑ Outings
Bathing ❑ Tub ❑ Shower ❑ Bed		**Restorative Nursing Program** ❑ No ❑ Yes _____
Personal Hygiene		
Oral care ❑ Own teeth ❑ Dentures ❑ No teeth		
Dressing		

Immediate Needs Care Plan

Resident Name _____ Date of Problem _____

PROBLEM/NEED

_____

_____

_____

_____

Goals	Interventions/Approaches	Resp. Disc.

Target Date _____ Signature/Title of Care Plan Writer _____

❑ Physician notified _____ ❑ Next of Kin notified _____ ❑ Staff informed of plan
time   time

NURSE'S NOTES

_____

_____

_____

_____

_____

_____

_____

_____

_____

_____

_____

_____

Core Care Plan

Resident Name _____

RAPs/QI _____

Problem/Need	Goals	Interventions	Resp. Disc.

Target Date

_____ _____ _____ _____

The Big Book of Care Plans, Second Edition

Comprehensive Nurse's Summary

Directions: Review ADL Plan, episodic nurse's notes, and resident. Circle applicable item in each column. Additional info may be written in or referred elsewhere. The Nurse Aide should participate in completion.

Resident Name _____   Time Period for Review _____

Functional Area	Status	Care Plan	Additional Remarks
MENTAL STATUS Short-Term Memory intact: Yes No Makes decisions: All Some None Understands: All Some None	Same Improved Deteriorating	Maintained Modified Initiated Not applicable	
BEHAVIOR PROBLEMS None Present, usually easily altered Present, usually not easily altered	Same Improved Deteriorating	Maintained Modified Initiated Not applicable	❑ Behavior Plan in place and followed except as noted in chart
MOOD Pleasant or easily cheered Sad, anxious Presents as depressed	Same Improved Deteriorating	Maintained Modified Initiated Not applicable	❑ Antidepressants in use ❑ Other Psychoactive given
HYGIENE/GROOMING I S LA EA TD **BED MOBILITY** I S LA EA TD **TRANSFER** I S LA EA TD **AMBULATION** I S LA EA TD	Same Improved Deteriorating	Maintained Modified Initiated Not applicable	❑ Restorative Program in Place for _____
NUTRITION/HYDRATION Food intake usual for resident Fluid intake is adequate w/wo assist Weight Stable	Yes No Yes No Yes No	Maintained Modified Initiated Not applicable	❑ Restorative Program in Place for _____
BOWELS Continent Incontinent BM 2+/wk Constipated Impaction(s)	Same Improved Deteriorating	Maintained Modified Initiated Not applicable	❑ Restorative Program in Place
BLADDER Continent Incontinent: occ freq always	Same Improved Deteriorating	Maintained Modified Initiated Not applicable	❑ Continence Management Program in place and followed
SKIN Intact Rash Bruise(s) Tear(s) Abrasion Cuts Burns **PRESSURE ULCER:** New Existing	Same Improved Deteriorating	Maintained Modified Initiated Not applicable	
FALLS No Yes Serious injury More than one occurrence	Same Improved Deteriorating	Maintained Modified Initiated Not applicable	
INFECTION(s) No Yes: UTI URI Pneu Skin Other	Same Improved Deteriorating	Maintained Modified Initiated Not applicable	

Interdisciplinary Team Progress Report

Resident Name _____ **Date** _____

Type of Review: Medicare Day: ❑ 5 ❑ 14 ❑ 30 ❑ 60 ❑ 90 ❑ OMRA ❑ Admission ❑ Quarterly ❑ Significant Change ❑ Annual ❑ Other

Quality Indicators that Triggered this Review and Explanation of Relationships/Causes

❑ New Fractures	❑ B&B HR	❑ Fecal Impaction	❑ Dehydration	❑ Psych med HR	❑ Restraints
❑ Falls	❑ B&B LR	❑ UTI	❑ Bedfast	❑ Psych med LR	❑ Little No Activity
❑ HR Behavior	❑ No Toilet Plan	❑ Weight Loss	❑ ADL	❑ Anti-Anxiety	❑ Pressure Ulcer HR
❑ LR Behavior	❑ Catheters	❑ Tube Feeding	❑ ROM	❑ Hypnotic	❑ Pressure Ulcer LR
❑ Depression					
❑ NO RX					
❑ 9+meds					
❑ Cognitive					

❑ If admit, significant change or annual review, Triggered RAPs with Indications for Care Planning

❑ Delirium	❑ ADL/Rehab	❑ Behavior	❑ Nutritional Status	❑ Dental
❑ Cognitive Loss/Dementia	❑ Incontinence/Catheter	❑ Restraints	❑ Feeding Tubes	❑ Pressure Ulcer
❑ Vision	❑ Psychosocial Well Being	❑ Activities	❑ Dehydration/Fluid Maintenance	❑ Psychotropic Drug Use
❑ Communication	❑ Mood	❑ Falls		

Immediate-Need Care Plan Patterns/Trends If applicable this review

_____
_____
_____
_____

Diagnosis

_____
_____
_____
_____

Directions: Begin by summarizing the resident's status inclusive of Quality Indicators triggered and clinical relationships of the indicators to each other if present. If an admission, significant change or annual review, note the causal relationships of RAPs to each other, with indications for Care Planning.

Include: Summary of Status,   QI Clinical Relationships,   RAP Clinical Relationships

_____
_____
_____
_____
_____
_____
_____
_____
_____
_____
_____
_____
_____
_____
_____

Interdisciplinary Team Progress Report (cont.)

STATUS OF CORE CARE PLAN GOALS AND MODIFICATIONS/ADDITIONS

Goal codes: **A** = Goal met—discontinue plan   **B** = Goal Met—continue plan for maintenance   **C** = Goal not met—plan revised/adjusted

Problem/Need Area or Plan Number	Goal status	Rationale for Actions/Plan Changes/Additions (if other than goal met, discontinue plan)

CARE PLAN, CONFERENCE, AND DISCUSSION ATTENDED BY AND/OR INCLUDED

Facility Personnel Signature	Discipline	❑ Resident ❑ Family ❑ Next of kin ❑ Significant other
		❑ Provided input prior to conference.
		❑ Unable to attend, report mailed post-conference.
		❑ Reviewed verbally post-conference with _____
		❑ Resident unable ❑ No interested parties
		❑ Attended, Signature below

Quality Indicator Incontinence Worksheet

Directions: Use the Resident-Level Summary Report to identify residents falling into categories, then determine what put them there and resident's ability to cooperate with toileting. Use the UI RAP and staff input to address other listed data.

Risk-adjusted Resident **Frequently Incontinent**	Mobility Dependent	Severe Cognitive Impairment	Additional Reasons	**Can Cooperate** Initiate Toilet Program		**Cannot cooperate** Initiate Check and Change Program	Comments
				Habit	Scheduled		

Risk-adjusted Resident **Always Incontinent**	Mobility Dependent	Severe Cognitive Impairment	Additional Reasons	**Can Cooperate** Initiate Toilet Program		**Cannot cooperate** Initiate Check and Change Program	Comments
				Habit	Scheduled		

Resident **Occasionally Incontinent Without Toileting Plan**	Voiding Pattern Present	Can Cooperate	Toileting Program Indicated				Type of Incontinence				
			H	P	S	None	Stress	Urge	Overflow Or Obstructive	Functional	Neurogenic

Resident **Frequently Incontinent Without Toileting Plan**	Voiding Pattern Present	Can Cooperate	Toileting Program Indicated				Type of Incontinence				
			H	P	S	None	Stress	Urge	Overflow Or Obstructive	Functional	Neurogenic

Habit = cooperative, without a voiding pattern.

Prompted = cooperative, can mobilize under own power, some awareness of bladder fullness.

Scheduled = cooperative, needs help to mobilize, pattern present.

Stress: small amounts, spurts

Urge: abrupt loss

Overflow/obstructive: dribble

Functional: physical, mental, psychosocial

Quality Indicator Behavior Symptoms Worksheet

Directions: Using the Resident-Level Summary Report, identify residents falling into high/low groups, then determine what put them there. Using the MDS and staff, determine alterability, use of psych meds, and symptoms exhibited.

MDS Symptoms Key: Physical Verbal Disruptive Inappropriate Social Behavior

High-Risk Resident	Cognitive Impairment	Psyhotic Disorders	Manic Depression	Behavior Easily Altered	Psychoactive Medication in Use	MDS Symptoms Noted				Comments
						P	V	D	I	

Low-Risk Resident	Reason or Problem Related to Symptoms		Behavior Easily Altered	Psychoactive Medication in Use	MDS Symptoms Noted				Comments
					P	V	D	I	

General Guidelines for Assessment and Documentation

- Cognitive Impairment with psychoactive med = CFR guidelines indicate behavior must be harmful to self, others, or so distressing resident is unable to function. If this is the case, clearly validate via document. If it is not the case, action must be initiated to reassess appropriateness.

- Psychoactive medication use if behavior not easily altered = review for length of time receiving, dosage, appropriateness.

- Psychoactive medication use if behavior is easily altered = review length of time receiving, appropriateness, continued need.

- If behavior is not easily altered always ask why, what are causes; look holistically.

- If behavior is easily altered always ask if it creates problems for resident or a problem in the environment. If so, care planning is indicated.

Quality Indicator Pressure Ulcer Worksheet

Directions: Use the Resident-Level Summary Report to identify resident category. Next, using the MDS, determine the risk factors that placed resident in the category. Note if improving or deteriorating, where developed, and avoidability if developed in house.

High-Risk Resident	Impaired Mobility	Impaired Transfer	Comatose	Mal-nutrition	End-Stage Disease	Acquired		Healing		Comments
						IN NF	Out NF	Yes	No	

Low-Risk Resident	Note any clinical conditions contributing to occurrence	Acquired		Healing		Comments
		IN NF	Out NF	Yes	No	

General Guidelines for Assessment and Documentation

Clinical conditions that can contribute to occurrence:

Continuous urinary incontinence or chronic voiding dysfunction; Chronic bowel incontinence; Severe peripheral vascular disease; Diabetes; desensitized skin, pitting edema, severe chronic pulmonary obstructive disease; Sepsis; Chronic renal, liver, and/or heart disease; disease or drug-related immunosuppression; full-body cast; Steroid therapy; Radiation therapy; Chemotherapy; Renal dialysis; or Head of bed elevated the majority of the day due to medical necessity.

Factors that can retard healing:

* Malnutrition/dehydration, whether secondary to poor appetite or another disease process, places resident at risk for poor healing.
* Clinical conditions above.
* Resident non-compliance with plan (note why and actions to address the problem).

In-house developed ulcers:

Documentation should reflect factors beyond facility control that resulted in occurrence of in-house pressure ulcers or that can account for lack of healing. Were risks identified? Was care plan initiated, followed, reviewed, and revised? If ulcer was potentially avoidable, documentation should reflect additional measures implemented to reverse the condition and prevent further occurrence. This may include more aggressive turning, positioning schedule, additional supplements, restorative programs, change in medication, and so on.

Non-healing ulcers:

Documentation should reflect factors that can account for lack of healing. Reflect on the clinical conditions that present that interfere with healing. Was the treatment plan for non-healing ulcers periodically reviewed and discussed with physician? Note documentation of rationale for not changing treatment plan after a reasonable period of time for non-healing ulcers.

The Big Book of Care Plans, Second Edition

Quality Indicator Depression Symptoms Worksheet

Directions: Using the Resident-Level Summary Report, identify residents with symptoms of depression. Determine alterability based on MDS, and note any use of psychoactive meds.

Resident Symptoms of Depression	Easily Cheered	Psychoactive Medication in Use				Comments
		AP	AA	Hypnotic	Antidepressant	

Resident Symptoms of Depression NO Anti-depressant Medication	Easily Cheered	Psychoactive Meds in Use			Comments
		AP	AA	Hypnotic	

General Guidelines for Assessment and Documentation

- If symptoms of depression, not easily cheered, and using anti-depressant, then evaluate med for length of time receiving, dosage, appropriateness, need for change.

- If symptoms of depression and receiving other class of psychoactive medication, consider possibility that this med may be a causative or contributing factor for symptoms. If not, be clear as to why medication is not a cause or contributor. If symptoms are NOT truly indicators of depression, then what underlying factors resulted in the items being noted on the MDS?

- If symptoms of depression, NOT easily cheered, and NO anti-depressant med given, evaluate symptoms and need for medication. If not indicated, be clear in your documentation as to why it would not be appropriate.

Quality Indicator Weight Loss Worksheet

Directions: Identify the residents with significant weight loss and the area(s) of impact, if any. Identify causative factors and document these facts in the clinical record, adjusting care plan as needed. Facility-based issues need to be addressed as a QA activity.

| Weight Loss Resident Name | Unplanned or Unexpected | | Impact/Outcome | | | | Causative factors | | |
	NO	YES	Pressure ulcers	Falls	Dehydration	ADL or ROM decline	Resident-based clinical condition (specify)	Facility-based	Unknown

Quality Indicator ADL Decline Worksheet

Directions: Identify the residents who triggered ADL decline and note any risk factors present. Note if restorative programming is in place, identifying if goals were maintenance, improvement, slowing decline, or lessening complications. Identify causative factors, actions, and correlations. Document these facts in the clinical record, adjusting care plan as needed.

ADL Decline Resident Name	Expected		High Risk Conditions Present				Restorative Program in Place		Comments
			Weight loss	Terminal end-stage	Decline in cognitive status	New acute condition			
	NO	YES					NO	YES	

Encyclopedia of Care Planning

Steps to Effective Care Planning

1. Complete professional assessments, including focused reviews on high-risk areas.

2. Initiate immediate need care planning. This care plan addresses the key needs to meet standards of care and practice.

3. Implement tracking tools to ensure accurate responses on the Minimum Data Set (MDS). At a minimum, track the late loss activities of daily living (ADLs) of bed mobility, eating, transfer, toileting, and mood/behavior.

4. Complete the MDS. Be sure you have consensus by having EACH discipline review the completed document prior to locking.

5. Complete and analyze the triggered resident assessment protocols (RAPs). This entails a review of the RAP guidelines, NOT just restating MDS triggering items.

6. Develop a worksheet for care planning: Identify the problems that need to be addressed, and how the problems relate to one another. It's like a grocery list you take to the store when you do your shopping, so you get all you need and don't overspend. This includes a review of the relationships between diagnosis, triggered RAPs, Quality Indicators, and resident strengths.

7. As a team (this means effective care conferencing), agree to care planning components:

    - Problems need identification: resident strengths, scope, severity, and stability of problems

    - Goal suitability and appropriateness

- Interventions to be employed

- Timelines for meeting the goals and/or evaluating the plan's effectiveness

- Primary discipline for monitoring and overseeing plan effectiveness

8. Ensure resident or surrogate decision-maker is in agreement with the plan.

9. Educate caregivers on plan.

10. Monitor plan implementation and effectiveness, modifying if need be.

11. Reevaluate plan according to established goal dates or as needs of the resident dictate.

- Met goals—Can the plan be discontinued? If not, why not?

- Unmet goals—Why wasn't the goal met? Problem over/underestimated, inadequately developed or off target? Inadequate time to meet? Goal too ambitious? Goal too ambiguous? Interventions not working? Interventions not consistently implemented? Resident not willing?

Critical Questions for Care Planning, Compliance, and Quality Outcomes

1. Is the care plan oriented toward preventing avoidable declines?

2. How does the care plan manage risk factors?

3. Does the care plan build on resident strengths?

4. Does the plan reflect standards of current professional practice?

5. Are there measurable goals and treatment outcomes?

6. Is the resident or surrogate involved? Have wishes been honored? Has sufficient information been given so that an informed choice can be made?

7. If resident refuses treatment, does the plan reflect alternative means to address the problem?

8. Is IDT expertise used to develop the plan?

9. How does the staff involve the resident or surrogate in care planning?

10. Are assessment and care planning needs met for new residents prior to MDS completion?

11. Are direct-care staff members informed and knowledgeable about the care planning goals and interventions?

General Care Planning Areas

I. Functional status. Compromise will result in some type of care planning dependent on where and how it impacts the person. This is a primary function of the RAPs.

II. Rehab and restorative nursing. Includes potential for improvement, maintenance, slowing of decline, and management of complication risk factors.

III. Health maintenance. Monitoring stable and unstable conditions and disease processes. Listing problems that no longer affect the resident, are controlled, or no longer need monitoring is a team decision based on how the problem affects the overall functioning or well being of the person.

IV. Discharge potential. Needs to be assessed at admission, annually, and as needed. Focus should center on what needs to happen before the person can be safely discharged and/or adjustment problems related to not being able to be discharged.

V. Medications. Medications can be an intervention for a problem or can be a problem in and of themselves. For example, the use of an antipsychotic may be an appropriate intervention to treat a schizophrenic, or it may have been inappropriately prescribed and require reduction and elimination and/or may be producing troubling side effects.

VI. Daily care needs. Standard practice approaches need not be placed on a care plan, particularly if they are expected facility actions. Daily care needs that are specific to the resident and are out of the ordinary must be addressed on the care plan.

Federal Certification Requirements and Guidelines for Care Planning

Federal Regulatory Requirement

Refer to F-Tag #272 §483.20: <u>Resident Assessment.</u>

To provide the facility with ongoing assessment information necessary to develop a care plan, to provide the appropriate care and services for each resident, and to modify the care plan and care/services based on the resident's status.

The facility is expected to use resident observation and communication as the primary source of information when completing the RAI. In addition to direct observation and communication with the resident, the facility should use a variety of other sources, including communication with licensed and non-licensed staff members on all shifts and may include discussions with the resident's physician, family members, or outside consultants and review of the resident's record.

F-Tag #271 (a) <u>Admission Orders.</u>

At the time each resident is admitted, the facility must have physician orders for the resident's immediate care.

§483.20(a) <u>Guidelines:</u>

"Physician orders for immediate care" are those written orders facility staff need to provide essential care to the resident, consistent with the resident's mental and physical status upon admission. These orders should, at a minimum, include dietary, drugs (if necessary), and routine care to maintain or improve the resident's functional abilities until staff can conduct a comprehensive assessment and develop an inter-disciplinary care plan.

F-Tag #272 (b) Comprehensive Assessments.

(1) Resident Assessment Instrument. A facility must make a comprehensive assessment of a resident's needs, using the RAI specified by the State. The assessment must include at least the following:

§483.20(b) Intent:

To ensure that the RAI is used in conducting comprehensive assessments as part of an ongoing process through which the facility identifies the resident's functional capacity and health status.

§483.20(b) Guidelines:

The facility is responsible for addressing all needs and strengths of residents regardless of whether the issue is included in the MDS or RAPs. The scope of the RAI does not limit the facility's responsibility to assess and address all care needed by the resident.

Furthermore, the facility is responsible for addressing the resident's needs from the moment of admission.

"Documentation of summary information (xvii) regarding the additional assessment performed through the resident assessment protocols (RAPs)" corresponds to MDS v. 2.0 Section V, and refers to documentation concerning which RAPs have been triggered, documentation of assessment information in support of clinical decision-making relevant to the RAP, documentation regarding where, in the clinical record, information related to the RAP can be found, and for each triggered RAP, whether the identified problem was included in the care plan.

(xviii) Documentation of participation in assessment.

"Documentation of participation in the assessment" corresponds to MDS v. 2.0 Section R, and refers to documentation of who participated in the assessment process. The assessment process must include direct observation and communication with the resident, as well as communication with licensed and non-licensed direct care staff members on all shifts.

F273 (2) *when required*. A facility must conduct a comprehensive assessment of a resident as follows:

(i) Within 14 calendar days after admission, excluding readmissions in which there is no significant change in the resident's physical or mental condition. (For purposes of this section, "readmission" means a return to the facility following a temporary absence for hospitalization or for therapeutic leave.)

<u>§483.20(b)(2) Intent:</u>

To assess residents in a timely manner.

F274 (ii) Within 14 days after the facility determines, or should have determined, that there has been a significant change in the resident's physical or mental condition. (For purpose of this section, a "significant change" means a major decline or improvement in the resident's status that will not normally resolve itself without further intervention by staff or by implementing standard disease-related clinical interventions, that has an impact on more than one area of the resident's health status, and requires interdisciplinary review or revision of the care plan, or both.)

<u>§483.20(b)(2)(ii) Guidelines:</u>

The following are the criteria for significant changes:

A significant change reassessment is generally indicated if decline or improvement is consistently noted in two or more areas of decline or two or more areas of improvement:

<u>Decline:</u>

- Any decline in activities of daily living (ADL) physical functioning where a resident is newly coded as 3, 4 or 8 Extensive assistance, Total dependency, Activity did not occur (note that even if coding in both columns A and B of an ADL category changes, this is considered one ADL change);

- Increase in the number of areas where Behavioral Symptoms are coded as "not easily altered" (e.g., an increase in the use of code 1's for E4B);

- Resident's decision-making changes from 0 or 1, to 2 or 3;

- Resident's incontinence pattern changes from 0 or 1 to 2, 3, or 4, or placement of an indwelling catheter;

- Emergence of sad or anxious mood as a problem that is not easily altered;

- Emergence of an unplanned weight loss problem (5% change in 30 days or 10% change in 180 days);

 The Big Book of Care Plans, Second Edition

- Begin to use trunk restraint or a chair that prevents rising for a resident when it was not used before;

- Emergence of a condition/disease in which a resident is judged to be unstable;

- Emergence of a pressure ulcer at Stage II or higher, when no ulcers were previously present at Stage II or higher; or

- Overall deterioration of resident's condition; resident receives more support (e.g., in ADLs or decision-making).

Improvement:

- Any improvement in ADL physical functioning where a resident is newly coded as 0, 1, or 2 when previously scored as a 3, 4, or 8;

- Decrease in the number of areas where Behavioral Symptoms or Sad or Anxious Mood are coded as "not easily altered;"

- Resident's decision making changes from 2 or 3, to 0 or 1;

- Resident's incontinence pattern changes from 2, 3, or 4 to 0 or 1; or

- Overall improvement of resident's condition; resident receives fewer supports.

If the resident experiences a significant change in status, the next annual assessment is not due until 366 days after the significant change reassessment has been completed.

F-Tag #278 (g) Accuracy of Assessment. The assessment must accurately reflect the resident's status.

(h) Coordination. A registered nurse must conduct or coordinate each assessment with the appropriate participation of health professionals.

(i) Certification.

    (1) A registered nurse must sign and certify that the assessment is completed.

    (2) Each individual who completes a portion of the assessment must sign and certify the accuracy of that portion of the assessment.

(j) Penalty for falsification.

    (1) Under Medicare and Medicaid, an individual who willfully and knowingly—

        (i) Certifies a material and false statement in a resident assessment is subject to a civil money penalty of not more than $1,000 for each assessment; or

        (ii) Causes another individual to certify a material and false statement in a resident assessment is subject to a civil money penalty or not more than $5,000 for each assessment.

(2) Clinical disagreement does not constitute a material and false statement.

§483.20(g) Intent:

To assure that each resident receives an accurate assessment by staff that are qualified to assess relevant care areas and knowledgeable about the resident's status and needs.

§483.20(g) Guidelines:

"The accuracy of the assessment" means that the appropriate, qualified health professional correctly documents the resident's medical, functional, and psychosocial problems and identifies resident strengths to maintain or improve medical status, functional abilities, and psychosocial status.

The initial comprehensive assessment provides baseline data for ongoing assessment of resident progress.

§483.20(h) Intent:

The registered nurse will conduct and/or coordinate the assessment, as appropriate. Whether conducted or coordinated by the registered nurse, he or she is responsible for certifying that the assessment has been completed.

§483.20(h) Guidelines:

According to the Utilization Guidelines for each state's RAI, the physical, mental, and psychosocial condition of the resident determines the appropriate level of involvement of physicians, nurses, rehabilitation therapists, activities professionals, medical social workers, dietitians, and other professionals, such as developmental disabilities specialists, in assessing the resident. Involvement of other disciplines is dependent upon resident status and needs.

§483.20(g)(h) Probes:

- Have appropriate health professionals assessed the resident? For example, has the resident's nutritional status been assessed by someone who is knowledgeable in nutrition and capable of correctly assessing a resident?

- If the resident's medical status, functional abilities, or psychosocial status declined and the decline was not clinically unavoidable, were the appropriate health professionals involved in assessing the resident?

- Based on your total review of the resident, is each portion of the assessment accurate?

F279 (k) Comprehensive Care Plans.

(1) The facility must develop a comprehensive care plan for each resident that includes measurable objectives and timetables to meet a resident's medical, nursing, and mental and psychosocial needs as identified in the comprehensive assessment. The care plan must describe the following:

> An interdisciplinary team, in conjunction with the resident, resident's family, surrogate, or representative, as appropriate, should develop quantifiable objectives for the highest level of functioning the resident may be expected to attain, based on the comprehensive assessment. The interdisciplinary team should show evidence in the RAP summary or clinical record of the following:

    – The resident's status in triggered RAP areas;

    – The facility's rationale for deciding whether to proceed with care planning; and

    – Evidence that the facility considered the development of care planning interventions for all RAPs triggered by the MDS.

The care plan must reflect intermediate steps for each outcome objective if identification of those steps will enhance the resident's ability to meet his or her objectives. Facility staff will use these objectives to monitor resident progress.

Facilities may, for some residents, need to prioritize their care plan interventions. This should be noted in the clinical record or on the plan of care.

- Does the care plan address the needs, strengths, and preferences identified in the comprehensive resident assessment?

- Is the care plan oriented toward preventing avoidable declines in functioning or functional levels? How does the care plan attempt to manage risk factors? Does the care plan build on resident strengths?

- Does the care plan reflect standards of current professional practice?

- Do treatment objectives have measurable outcomes?

- Corroborate information regarding the resident's goals and wishes for treatment in the plan of care by interviewing residents, especially those identified as refusing treatment.

- Determine whether the facility has provided adequate information to the resident so that the resident was able to make an informed choice regarding treatment.

- If the resident has refused treatment, does the care plan reflect the facility's efforts to find alternative means to address the problem?

<u>§483.20(k)(2) Probes:</u>

1. Was interdisciplinary expertise utilized to develop a plan to improve the resident's functional abilities?

    a. For example, did occupational therapist design needed adaptive equipment, or did speech therapist provide techniques to improve swallowing ability?

    b. Do the dietitian and the speech therapist determine, for example, the optimum textures and consistency for the resident's food that provide both a nutritionally adequate diet and effectively use oropharyngeal capabilities of the resident?

    c. Is there evidence of physician involvement in development of the care plan (e.g., presence at care planning meetings, conversations with team members concerning the care plan, conference calls)?

2. In what ways do staff members involve residents and families, surrogates, and/or representatives in care planning?

3. Do staff members make an effort to schedule care plan meetings at the best time of the day for residents and their families?

4. Ask the ombudsman if he/she has been involved in a care planning meeting as a resident advocate. If yes, ask how the process worked.

5. Do facility staff attempt to make the process understandable to the resident/family?

6. Ask residents whether they have brought questions or concerns about their care to the attention of facility staff. If so, what happened as a result?

7. Is the care plan evaluated and revised as the resident's status changes?

(i) Meet professional standards of quality and;

"Professional standards of quality" means services that are provided according to accepted standards of clinical practice. Standards may apply to care provided by a particular clinical discipline or in a specific clinical situation or setting. Standards regarding quality care practices may be published by a professional organization, licensing board, accreditation body, or other regulatory agency. Possible reference sources for standards of practice include:

- Current manuals or textbooks on nursing, social work, physical therapy, etc.

- Standards published by professional organizations such as the American Dietetic Association, American Medical Association, American Medical Directors Association, American Nurses Association, National Association of Activity Professionals, National Association of Social Work, etc.

- Clinical-practice guidelines published by the Agency of Health Care Policy and Research.

- Current professional journal articles.

If a negative resident outcome is determined to be related to the facility's failure to meet professional standards, and the team determines a deficiency has occurred, it should be cited under the appropriate quality-of-care or other relevant requirement.

§483.20(k)(3) Probes:
Question only those practices which have a negative outcome or have a potential negative outcome. Ask the facility to produce references upon which the practice is based.

1. Do nurses notify physicians as appropriate, and show evidence of discussions of acute medical problems?

2. Are residents promptly hospitalized when they have acute conditions that require intensive monitoring and hospital-level treatments that the facility is unable to provide?

3. Are there errors in the techniques of medication administration? (Cite actual medication errors at §483.25(m).)

4. Is there evidence of assessment and care planning sufficient to meet the needs of newly admitted residents prior to completion of the first comprehensive assessment and comprehensive care plan?

5. Physicians' orders carried out, unless otherwise indicated by an advanced directive?

F282 (ii) Be provided by qualified persons in accordance with each resident's written plan of care.

<u>§483.20(k)(3)(ii) Guidelines:</u>

If you find problems with quality of care, quality of life, or resident rights, are these problems attributable to the qualifications of the facility staff, or lack of, inadequate, or incorrect implementation of the care plan?

Can direct caregiving staff describe the care, services, and expected outcomes of the care they provide, have a general knowledge of the care and services being provided by other therapists, have an understanding of the expected outcomes of this care, and understand the relationship of these expected outcomes to the care they provide?

Essential Assessments for On-Target Care Plans

The Minimum Data Set 2.0

The MDS acts as a general quality assurance check on the resident's functional status. It provides a holistic picture of the resident's status. Consequently, all caregivers must be involved in the process. Supporting documentation is generally indicated to validate MDS coding.

The MDS requires information to be collected from different time periods over the last seven, 14, 30, 60, and 90 days, and in some instances the last 120 days.

Resident Assessment Protocols

The care planning process begins with professional assessments. Nursing initiates the process at the time of admission continuing the process throughout the resident's stay. Shortly after admission social services, dietary, and activities begin their review and evaluation of the residents. These professional assessments lay the groundwork for the comprehensive assessment, which consists of the MDS and RAPs. Therapy may be involved in the assessment and care planning process from the outset or may be brought on board as the assessment process unfolds or as a resident changes.

The MDS identifies actual and potential problem areas that require further evaluation and investigation. These are referred to as "triggers." These triggers begin the specific analysis, an in-depth review of the related RAP. Wrong or lacking information regarding either results in inadequate care planning.

The RAPs provide the definitive analysis. There are four types of RAP triggers. Determining the type of trigger provides a better perspective on what to look for and how to think about the area under review.

1. **Broad Screening** triggers are designed to identify hard-to-diagnose problems. These include the delirium and dehydration RAPs.

2. **Rehabilitative Potential** triggers are geared to identify residents who may have rehab potential. Some items trigger because they indicate strengths that can be used to offset and/or assist in working through problems. The ADL, psychosocial well being and communication, cognitive loss, feeding tubes, and urinary incontinence RAPs are possible examples of these.

RAP Principle

1. No RAP has been reviewed without considering the guidelines contained in the RAP.

2. Collecting and recording data is the beginning of RAP review.

3. RAP review is completed when information has been analyzed and care planning decisions validated.

3. **Potential Problem** triggers determine if underlying issues are present that increase risk for negative outcomes. Pressure ulcers, feeding tubes, restraints, urinary incontinence, mood, behavior, psychoactive drug, dental, and activity RAPs are potential examples of these.

4. **Prevention of Problem** triggers alert the staff to presence of risk factors and potential complications. These might include the cognitive loss, mood, behavior, restraints, vision, fall, pressure ulcer, or urinary incontinence RAPs.

How to get the best results with RAPs

There is no mandated method. The facility needs to consider the best options for their circumstances. Here are some recommendations for "best" results and greatest efficiency of data collection:

- Combine RAP guidelines in professional assessments. It is possible to capture 11 RAPs in this manner. You get a more comprehensive assessment and avoid duplication of effort if the RAPs trigger. On the RAP summary sheet indicate location of information as the professional assessment(s).

- Use risk assessment tools for specific problem-prevention RAPs. Consider fall- and skin-risk assessments as "always" RAPs.

- Complete RAPs as they become evident, particularly those that can create negative outcomes and regulatory headaches. These include restraints, psychoactive drugs, and incontinence.

- The ADL RAP will always trigger unless the person is independent. The sooner you evaluate, the better the outcome and potential impact on case-mix scores.

Quality measure/quality indicator reports

The MDS also generates Quality Measure/Quality Indicator (QM/QI) reports. Quality Measures/Quality Indicators are used by the state surveyors to identify potential care problems in the facility. Since the information for the QM/QIs comes directly from the MDS, inaccurate QM/QIs can create problems on survey.

Surveyors will actually target residents they want to look at PRIOR to coming to the facility and will also determine how and where they will focus their time in the facility. Accurate coding and solid supporting documentation is the facility's only protection.

Using the **Resident-Level Summary** generated by the Quality Measures/Quality Indicators as part of the care planning process can act as the stamp of approval on the care plans created. The summary report enables the reviewer to critically evaluate the cause-and-effect relationship of triggered measures/indicators. The resident's triggered QM/QIs should be reviewed and discussed at each care conference and compared to the care plan developed or being created.

If your software cannot create the measure/indicator reports prior to locking the MDS you can determine them manually if you know what MDS items trigger the Quality Measure/Quality Indicators (a simple and quickly assimilated task).

Keep in mind that surveyors will be using the QM/QIs. It stands to reason, that if a QM/QI triggers, the surveyor will be looking for the related care plan or some pretty substantive documentation as to why care planning has not been indicated.

Comparison of RAPs to Quality Measures/Quality Indicators

The 18 Resident Assessment Protocols		The 24 Quality Indicators	
Delirium	Activities	New Fractures	Weight Loss
Cognitive Loss	Falls	Falls	Tube feedings
Visual Function	Nutritional Status	Behavior (high and low risk)	Dehydration
Communication	Feeding Tubes	Depression	Bedfast
ADL Function	Dehydration/Fluid Maintenance	Depression without use of antidepressant	ADL Decline
Urinary Incontinence/Catheters	Oral/Dental care	9+med use	Decline in ROM
Psychosocial Well Being	Pressure Ulcers	Incidence of Cognitive Impairment	Psychotropic Drug High and low risk
Mood	Psychotropic Drugs	B&B Incontinence (high and low risk)	Anti-anxiety
Behavioral Symptoms	Physical Restraints	Incontinence without Toileting Plan	Hypnotic
		Indwelling catheters	Restraints
		Fecal Impaction	Little/No Activity
			Pressure Ulcers

Resident Quality Measures/Quality Indicators Worksheet

Directions: Note resident name and review date then check off the indicators that triggered for the resident. Review these triggered indicators as part of your care plan review to validate that appropriate care planning has taken place.

Name										
Date										
New fractures										
Falls										
Behavior symptoms										
Symptoms of depression										
Depression with No TX										
9 + meds										
Incidence cognitive impairment										
Freq/always incontinent										
Occ/freq incont. with no toileting plan										
Indwelling catheter										
Fecal impaction										
UTI last 30 days										
Weight loss										
Tube feed										
Dehydration										
Bedfast										
Decline in late loss ADL										
Decline in ROM/increased functional limitation										
Antipsychotic use absent of psychotic/related condition										
Anti-anxiety/hypnotic use										
Hypnotic use two or more days in last week										
Daily use of physical restraints										
Little or no activity										
Pressure ulcers stage 1 to 4										

Suggested Best Practices for MDS Supporting Documentation

MDS 2.0 section critical areas	Time period	Suggested method for caputuring data	What you are looking for

E1 Mood Indicators
    Code 1 = up to 5 days
    Code 2 = 6, 7 days / >
	Last 30 Days
	
	Last 90 Days
		Nurse's Comprehensive Summary Notes
		Social Service and Activity Periodic Assessments
		Seven-Day Mood and Behavior Tracker
			Occurrence
			
			Change in status

E2 Mood Persistence	Last 7 Days	Seven-Day Mood and Behavior Tracker	Alterability

E4 Behavior Symptoms
    Code 1 = 1-3 days
    Code 2 = 4-6 days
    Code 3 = daily or more
	Last 7 Days
	
	Last 90 Days
		Seven-Day Mood and Behavior Tracker
		Nurse's Comprehensive Summary
		Social Service and Activity Periodic Assessments
			Frequency and Alterability
			Change in status

G Physical Function **Critical:** Bed Mobility, Eating, Toilet Use, Transfer **Non-critical:** Walking in room/ corridor; Locomotion on and off unit; Dressing, Personal Hygiene	Last 7 Days Last 90 Days	Seven-Day ADL Tracker Nurse's Comprehensive Summary	Average ADL self performance Most amount of staff support provided Change in status
H Continence	Last 14 Days Last 90 Days	Bowel Movement Flow Record Urinary Incontinence POC and Nurse's Notes (Periodic or Comprehensive) Nurse's Comprehensive Summary	Frequency of Self-controlled or incontinence Change in status

K   Oral/Nutrition
    Nutritional problems
 	
    Parenteral or enteral intake
	Last 7 Days
	
	Last 7 Days
		Seven-Day ADL Tracker
		
		Medication/treatment record
			Amount of intake
			Food complaints

N Activity Pursuits Time awake Time Involved Activities	Last 7 Days Morning 7–12 Afternoon 12–5 Evening 5–10	Seven-Day Mood and Behavior Tracker Activity Assessment Last 90 days Activity Assessment	Naps no more than one hour per time period. Time spent pursuing interest. Change in status Required by HCFA MDS
Pib Therapy	Last 7 Days 15 minutes or >/Day	Physician orders, evaluation, plan, program delivery records, and progress notes	Required by HCFA MDS Supporting documentation to validate MDS, RUGs
P3 Restorative Nursing	Last 7 Days 15 minutes or >	Evaluation and POC goals and interventions Delivery records and periodic progress notes	As above

Evaluating and Acting on Triggered Quality Indicators

New fractures: Review for potential relationship to falls, behavior, and incontinence.

1. Fractures occurring outside the facility or prior to admission need to be reviewed. When possible identify potential for like circumstances that could occur in the facility, address accordingly in the assessment and care plan.

2. Fracture that occurs while in facility: review clinical record for determination of avoidability.

    • Check record for assessment/evaluation of causative factors. If none present, review status and make entry addressing the reevaluation and any additional plans.

    • Review care plans for presence, appropriateness, and need for modification.

Falls: Review relationship with incontinence, psychoactive meds, behavior, depression, weight loss, and dehydration.

1. Identify residents with both falls and new fracture. Record must aggressively address plan to minimize re-occurrence. If clinically unavoidable, document why.

2. Review each resident listed for cluster falls. That is, more than one has occurred in the last month or quarter.

    • Was the resident appropriately assessed? Is an at-risk plan in place? Has it been modified since falls? If not, why not? Is this an isolated case or are patterns present in the facility? If so, initiate QA activities immediately to define causative factors and corrective actions.

    • Resident-based causes: If no modification to the plan is needed, be sure to clearly document review of the plan with each fall and why the plan remains appropriate. Be sure the plan goal is not "will not fall" on these residents. Rather, focus plan on minimizing risk for serious injury. Be sure that the clinical circumstances creating the unavoidability are clearly documented for each occurrence and easily located within the record.

Behavior/emotional patterns

High-risk behavior: Review relation potential to psychoactive medication, 9+ med use, incontinence, depression, and activities.

1.   Identify what criteria placed the resident in the high-risk group.

Cognitive impairment: any impairment in decision-making and short-term memory problems.

Resident-based/staff contributors and causes:

- Is behavior a catastrophic response (resident decompensates from lack of comprehension/ miscomprehension or inability to act on demands made on them)? If so, under what circumstances? (E.g., strikes out with hands on care attempts. Is this clearly outlined and specific interventions noted on care plan? Does behavior subside with planned/implemented interventions? If not, does the plan need to be altered or is additional staff training, counseling, or monitoring needed?)

- Is behavior unpredictable and not easily altered? Is it causing distress to the resident or others? Is the resident or are others at risk? Have non-medical interventions been implemented? If so, use of medication may be indicated.

- Are psychoactive meds used in response to outburst? Why? Is it a response to the episode or given proactively to minimize or prevent occurrence because of the distress it causes for the residents or to others? Would behavior subside on its own without medication?

- Does social services address the problem, including frequency, alterability, and severity? Is the effectiveness of the non-medical management plan addressed?

- Does activities have a structured program in place on a daily basis? If not, why?

- Is the rationale appropriate?

Psychotic disorder, schizophrenia, or manic depression

- Is psychoactive medication in use? Is it possible that medication side effects are responsible for behaviors? Consider discussing with pharmacist, then physician as appropriate.

The Big Book of Care Plans, Second Edition

- Is psychoactive medication effective? That is, functional status is same or better than prior to use AND without side effects. If no to either or both, initiate physician contact to address possible change in med regimen.

- Is there a non-medical management plan in place? Is it known? Is it followed consistently? Has it been or does it need to be reviewed or modified? If stated goals are not being met, care plan changes are indicated.

- Does social services address the problem and effectiveness of the non-medical management plan?

- Does activities have a structured program in place on a daily basis? If not, why? Is the rationale appropriate? Is it related to resident refusal, lifestyle choices, or lack of meaningful programming for the individual?

Low-risk behavior

- Is this a lifelong pattern? If so, has social services clearly addressed it as such?

- Does the care plan address the problem from a complication risk standpoint?

- Is the behavior related to clinical complications? If so, have nursing and social services clearly addressed it as such? Is the physician aware? Do progress notes reflect his or her awareness? Does the care plan address the behavior from a complication-risk standpoint?

- Is this behavior recent? Was it sporadic or of no consequence? If not, has it been assessed for causative factors, both psychosocial (e.g., depression, loss, boredom, etc.) and physical (e.g., pain, major disability, etc.). Has a care plan been created to focus on reversal or elimination of the problem, and/or complications and risk?

- Is this potentially or actually a significant status change? Is behavior easily altered?

- If not, why, and what additional actions might be needed?

- Evaluate from a facility perspective if above 50th – 75th percentile. What action or practices might be taking place that are creating the problems? For example, is activity programming adequate? Is the environment comfortable, and without annoyances and stressors such as buzzers and alarms sounding frequently?

Depression: Cross-check with falls, behavior, psychoactive meds, decline in ADL, weight loss, incontinence.

- Check each triggered resident. Are symptoms easily altered? Are symptoms lifelong or a change from "normal"?

- Are the symptoms affecting their well being, functional level, or health? If not, be sure the record demonstrates this. If so, are they receiving antidepressant medication?

- Residents on medication who continue to have symptoms of depression that are not easily altered or impacting negatively on their overall functional status need to be discussed with the physician. The care plan needs to reflect and address the complications and risk factors.

Depression without treatment

- If symptoms are easily altered (the resident is easily cheered) be sure the clinical record reflects this along with a care plan that addresses what the interventions are.

- If the resident is not easily cheered, is this a lifelong pattern of behavior? If so, be sure the documentation reflects this, and note if it presents any complications or risk factors for the individual. If it does, be sure the care plan addresses them accordingly. If it doesn't, an assessment note of explanation will be sufficient. However, as long as the symptoms are present it would be wise to make a periodic notation to this effect in conjunction with quarterly review.

- In the presence of symptoms that are not easily altered and impacting negatively on the resident's functional status, the use of antidepressant therapy should be considered. Is the physician aware? If the physician is aware and chooses not to treat with antidepressants, supporting documentation from the physician is indicated which addresses alternate treatment plans and/or complication risks present and how they will be managed.

Use of nine or more different medications

- As residents come up for quarterly review, request that the pharmacist specifically review residents' medication profiles in conjunction with their clinical status and presentation, as well as for potential duplicative drug side effects, particularly related to other QIs that have triggered for the individual. This will be most effective when done with the RN responsible for care.

- Have the Interdisciplinary Team discuss the medications and potential alternatives for decreasing use. Reflect the results of the discussion in the team notes.

Incidence of cognitive impairment: Cross-check with psychoactive meds and depression.

- If a true status change, can you pinpoint the cause? Was it insidious or rapid? Has it been evaluated for reversibility or accepted as inevitable (i.e. could there be a new or worsening depression)? Be sure the record clearly reflects identification of the problem and actions initiated. This should be done in conjunction with a significant status-change assessment, or episodically on noting the change in mental functioning in the absence of other overt conditions.

Elimination/Incontinence: Check the other QIs that triggered. Are there relationships with restraints, bedfast, decline ADL, ROM?

High-risk bowel or bladder incontinence. Identify what criteria placed the resident in the high-risk group.

Severe cognitive impairment. If the resident is cooperative and able to be mobilized, consider habit training. If not, establish a routine program for checking and changing. Be sure your care plan addresses complications and risks associated with this uncorrectable problem (e.g., behavior outburst, poor hygiene, UTI, etc.).

Total dependence in mobility. In the absence of severe cognitive impairment consider the reversibility or minimizing the degree of occurrence.

- Determine if external forces, policies, or practices such as the use of restraints and psychoactive meds are impacting on the resident's ability to mobilize.

- Think about the possibility of an aggressive restorative program to improve mobility status if not contraindicated for the individual.

- Review care plan. Is the staff implementing the plan consistently? Is the staff responsive and anticipating the need to toilet? If staffing is a problem, is there a system to prioritize care needs?

Occasional or frequent incontinence without a toileting plan: Cross-check for relationships to falls, psychoactive meds, pressure ulcers, behavior, depression, dehydration, and fecal impaction.

- Occasional or frequent incontinence suggests that something can be done to reverse and/or further minimize occurrence. You will need to evaluate your existing policies, practices, and staff attitudes about incontinence management. You may need to establish or update your program.

- For those who are only occasionally incontinent, determine if you can pinpoint these occurrences or if they are sporadic, with no predictability. If you can pinpoint, obviously you will build your care plan accordingly. If you cannot, then determine if the occasional incontinence creates risk for the individual and address as part of care planning. If risks are absent and/or minimal you can consider addressing rationale for no care planning in a progress or RAP note.

- For those who are frequently incontinent, the Incontinence RAP can be a major help. Focus on times when the person IS continent. Can you build on that? Review the information in the RAI manual in its entirety first. Then evaluate your current facility practices, taking action accordingly. It will be important to determine, if possible, the type of urinary incontinence the individual has. That information will improve the likelihood of lessening and/or reversing the problem.

Indwelling catheters: Cross-check to UTI, dehydration, and pressure ulcer QIs for possible correlation. Determine cause-effect scenario.

- What is the clinical reason for the catheter? Does it impact on functional status? If so, in what way? Is it addressed on the care plan? Could catheterization be intermittent rather than continuous? Why or why not? Include this in your medical record discussion of the problem/need. What are the complications/risks for this individual? How are they managed? Is the management effective?

Fecal impaction: Cross-check to dehydration, weight loss, and medications.

- If it is true impaction evaluate for causative factors.

    - Is it food-, fluid-, or mobility-related or exacerbated? What actions have or could be taken by the facility to improve this? If not, why not? Be sure the reasons are recorded in the medical record.

– Is it med related or exacerbated? If so, can a different med be substituted? If not, why not? Record in chart, as well as care plan complications/risks and interventions.

– Is it a result of disease process? If so, request that the physician address as such in progress notes periodically and/or summarize in your assessment notes. Care plan complications/ risks and interventions.

– Was the risk for impaction recognized? Was it care planned? If the goals were not met was resident reassessed and care plan revised?

Urinary tract infections: Cross-check with incontinence, catheters, and dehydration.

• Check medical record. Is there supporting documentation to indicate UTI did occur within 30 days of assessment reference date window?

• Does the chart support presence of a true UTI (i.e., positive cultures and symptoms were present)? If not, evaluate if this was an isolated issue or a systemic problem related to facility policies or practices, including the need for staff training.

• For each resident determine if UTIs are more than an isolated event. If so, have you evaluated the causes? Is it something you can reverse or minimize? Was care planning in place? Was it followed? Is revision needed?

• Review your infection control program for monitoring and investigating to be sure you are in compliance (i.e., tracking by site, source, organism, unit, caregivers, etc.).

Weight loss: Check for relationship to tube feedings, pressure ulcers, and ADL/ROM decline. Check each resident's record for accuracy of weights, avoidability, and current status.

• If weight loss was anticipated or intended, be sure the assessment and care plan reflect the why and how.

• If unintended, why did it occur? If it is a resident-based reason, be sure the circumstances surrounding the loss and the facility actions to address it are clearly documented. If a facility-based problem, determine the probable causes and check them out to be sure you aren't assuming. Once identified, implement a corrective action plan, re-study, and proceed accordingly.

Tube feedings: Check relationship to weight loss, ADL, cognitive decline.

- Review each resident for continuing need, presence of any side effects, and how they are managed.

- If resident is also receiving oral feedings, is there an aggressive plan in place to eliminate dependence on the tube feeding as primary source of nutrition? Be sure your documentation reflects why or why not.

Dehydration: Check for relationship to weight loss, ADL decline, cognitive decline, pressure ulcers, fecal impaction, UTI, restraints, and psychoactive drugs.

- Is dehydration valid based on the assessment reference date? Is there supporting documentation on record (e.g., fluid output exceeded fluid intake, symptoms present such as poor turgor, dry mucous membranes, etc.)? Was it unavoidable? Be sure the record clearly demonstrates this (such as MD note and/or your summary of factors indicating why).

- Is prevalence a result of a diagnosis that was not an active problem being coded on the MDS? If so, initiate staff training. Consider re-do of assessment for correction of miscoding.

Bedfast: Check relationship to activities, pressure ulcers, catheters, UTI, dehydration, weight loss, ADL decline, ROM decline, behavior, restraints.

- Was the MDS coded correctly? Check the MDS manual for the definition of bedfast.

- Is bedfast status appropriate? Be sure record is clear as to why or why not, what actions are in place to address it, and the complication risks.

- Are other QIs a cause or an outcome of being bedfast?

Decline in ADL: Check for potential relationships to weight loss, pressure ulcers, dehydration, incontinence, restraint, activities, drugs, cognition, bedfast.

- Was the decline related to an acute or unstable condition? Is it reversible? Is it clearly noted in the chart?

- Was it avoidable? If it was avoidable, what are the factors that created the situation? What is the incidence of occurrence compared to others? Are there problems within the care delivery system that need to be evaluated further (e.g., use and compliance with care plan, content of care plans, supervisions, etc.)?

- Was the occurrence a paper issue, not a real occurrence for the resident, based on a change of assessors? If so, evaluate your data collection system. A change in assessors should not result in a paper status decline if information is being sought from all sources across all shifts.

Decline in ROM: Check relationship to restraints, bedfast, ADL, cognition.

- Was the occurrence a paper issue, not a real occurrence for the resident, or based on a change of assessors? If so, evaluate your assessor's knowledge of evaluating status, including review of MDS criteria. If coded in error, consider doing a correction MDS.

- If decline is real, was it avoidable? Document the clinical factors and ensure the care plan addresses complications and risk.

- Too often, the decline was avoidable. What are the dynamics occurring in the facility. Is it a staffing shortage? Education or supervisory issue? Who is responsible for ensuring the interventions occur? Is it a paper oversight only? Identify all the possible reasons, and then review residents at risk and those with actual declines to determine causative factors.

Psychotropic drug use: Check the relationship to high- and low-risk behaviors, depression, depression without treatment, little/no activity, pressure ulcers, cognitive and ADL decline, incontinence, impaction, weight loss, falls.

High-risk antipsychotic

Determine if in this category because of cognitive impairment, diagnosis-based, or both.

Cognitive impairment

Is med use in response to behavior outbursts that are staff- or environmentally induced (refer to behavior indicator information)? These are facility-based problems that require further evaluation.

- Review orientation and ongoing training regarding care and interventions for cognitively impaired.

- Environmental evaluation for causes and contributors that may prompt or escalate behavior problems like overstimulation (too much activity, noise levels [like alarms]), or understimulation, such as lack of activity programming, sitting in a dark room, etc.

Is medication given related to symptoms that are creating frightful distress to self or others? These are resident-based needs/problems. Check that all appropriate actions have been taken by the facility.

- Are these symptoms identified and tracked?

- Is a behavior management program in place, followed, and reevaluated? Are these symptoms identified and tracked?

- Is the behavior easily altered with use of medication? If not, drug effectiveness and appropriateness need to be reassessed.

- Is the resident without adverse side effects from med? Compare to other indicators for possible relationship.

Psychotic disorder, manic depression

If the behavior is not easily altered you must evaluate two factors:

- Is a non-medical management plan in place, followed, and reevaluated for effectiveness?

- Is the medication not at a therapeutic dose or does a different medication need to be considered?

Low-risk antipsychotic

- Why is the medication being given? Does the resident have a condition that permits use of the medication? Is it clearly documented? Is the resident without adverse drug effects? Compare to other triggered indicators.

- If there is no valid clinical reason for use, can you trace the origin of the order and length of time receiving? Has a reduction/elimination program been tried and failed? If it failed, why? Was there a failure to create and implement a non-medical management plan?

- What is the need and reason for continued use? Is it possible the resident has a depression going on that has been missed and/or untreated?

Anti-anxiety: Correlate relationship to other triggered QIs: falls, behavior, depression, 9+ meds, incontinence, and ADL decline.

- If anti-anxiety is used routinely, why? Is this a resident demand? What attempts have been made to address this? Is there a risk plan in place?

- Is it clinically indicated? Is documentation in place? Are there adverse effects that can be tied to other triggered indicators? Is there a risk plan in place?

- If use is PRN, is it given proactively to facilitate treatment or calm in anticipation of predictable reaction? Is there a care plan in place for this? Is effectiveness noted?

- Is med used in response to behavior outburst or mood problem? Could that outburst have been anticipated and dealt with non-medically and/or proactively with medication? Is there a care plan in place? Is there documentation of need and interventions tried prior to administration? Is effectiveness noted? Is there monitoring for adverse effects?

Hypnotics and hypnotic use more than two times per week

- Evaluate the resident's sleep/wake cycle. Compare to MDS coding for time awake. Is it accurate? Check for correlation with depression, depression without treatment, behavior problems, little/no activity programming. To regulate sleep/wake cycle, typical use would be no more than 10 days (CFR criteria).

- Consider that you may have under-utilization as well as over-utilization. The average person, regardless of age needs six to eight hours of sleep. As you age, the quality of sleep diminishes.

  - A resident may be cat napping, collecting the sleep time they require during the day, resulting in use of hypnotic at night.

  - Lack of stimulation during the day can also contribute to sleep/wake problems. Check for possible correlation between sleep/wake cycle, hypnotic use, and activity programming.

  - Does the resident have pain? Is sleep disrupted? Would hypnotic enable or promote the resident to sleep? PRN is therapeutic dependent on resident clinical status.

Restraints: Correlate for possible relationships to falls, behavior, psychoactive med, 9+ meds, decline in ADL, ROM, cognition, weight loss, activities, pressure ulcers, incontinence.

- Is there a medical need present? Is it documented?

- Have risk factors been identified and care planned? Have they materialized (compare to other QIs)?

- Is there an aggressive activity program in pace? Is social services monitoring for adverse psychosocial impact? Is there an aggressive restorative program to ensure no related status decline occurs?

Little to no activity: Each resident with this QI needs to be reviewed to determine if the lack of programming is impacting negatively on the resident. Behavior, depression, cognitive impairment, and incontinence are potential major relationship players.

Pressure ulcers: Check for relationship to fractures, depression, weight loss, dehydration, psychoactive meds, 9+ meds, restraints, dehydration, bedfast, activities.

High risk:

Impaired transfer or bed mobility, comatose, malnutrition, or end-stage disease.

- Determine what placed the resident in a high-risk group and if risks noted were effectively managed. Was the ulcer clinically unavoidable? Is there documentation to support this belief?

Low risk:

Generally these ulcers are avoidable. If there are extenuating clinical circumstances, these must be clearly noted in the record. Physician documentation will be very helpful in addition to the IDT.

Putting the Care Plan Together

Writing problem statements

Decide if you are dealing with an issue or a problem. Problems are usually the outcome of those unsolvable issues. The RAPs and Quality Indicators will assist in this often complex task.

Issue: General statement that is past- or future oriented.

- Typically not solvable

- Almost impossible to develop measurable, achievable goals (i.e., confused and disoriented)

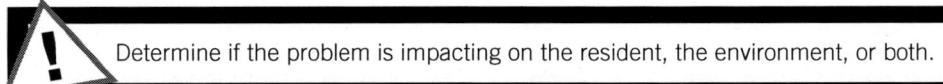

Determine if the problem is impacting on the resident, the environment, or both.

Problem: Specific statement that is here and now oriented.

- Typically the outcome or impact of the issue

- Goal development flows easily (i.e., confused and disoriented resulting in risk for weight loss from failure to feed self; and elopement attempts when seeking to "go to work")

Holistic thinking: As you identify the issue/problems ask yourself: What is this creating? How is this impacting or being demonstrated for this person physically, mentally, socially, and/or emotionally? Is it also impacting on the environment physically, mentally, socially, and/or emotionally?

Answering these questions gives you the care plan problem statement and enhances the quality of the goal(s) you write!

Developing goals

You will find it difficult, if not impossible, to develop measurable, doable, appropriate goals if your problem statement is addressing an issue instead of a problem. If there is ever any doubt about the level of goal development, always shoot for the highest goal first. You won't know if you don't try! Just be careful not to disable the resident or the team with unrealistic, unattainable goals.

There are five questions to ask to ensure a goal is in line with resident capabilities:

1. Is this solvable/fixable?

2. Is this something that might be improved?

3. Is this an area where maintenance is possible?

4. Can the decline be slowed?

5. Is there nothing that can be done to correct, reverse, or retard the problem? If the answer is yes, ask: What are the complications and risk factors attendant to this unfixable problem?

Goals must be measurable enough to readily identify if the plan is working. Avoid boxing yourself in. Don't hang yourself and make needless work when you don't have to. The best and easiest way to measure is by example—in other words, stated in action term or by observation.

Problem	Poor stamina requires one assist to ambulate. Is alert and motivated to improve function.	**Goal**	Will ambulate unassisted to and from bathroom.
Problem	Poor fluid intake, lacks initiative to drink, at risk for dehydration and UTI. Does respond to prompts given.	**Goal**	Will consume most liquids offered at meals and drink one cup fluid between breakfast, lunch, and dinner eliminating risk for dehydration and UTI. Or Will be free of dehydration and UTI as evidenced by soft bowel movement every three days, moist mouth, and clear to light colored urine.

The plan would go on to describe what actions to take if the goal was not met. For instance, providing foods high in water content, or alerting the nurse to take certain steps.

If there were a high risk of occurrence coupled with poor compliance, focused attention by the staff would be needed daily. If the probability of occurrence was low, but risk still a possible occurrence, the goal would be developed differently as noted in the second example.

Comparison of Care Plan Problem/Goal Statements

	NOT GOOD		BETTER
Problem	Depressed, makes negative self-statements	**Problem**	Exhibits depression as evidenced by: lack of attention to personal appearance, grooming, and negative self-statements about her appearance.
Comments	*So what if she makes negative self-statements? Lots of people do this and aren't necessarily depressed! This is a general statement that lacks substance. To move out of issue and care plan, you specifically need ask yourself what is being created HERE and NOW physically, mentally, socially, and emotionally for the resident and in the environment.* *How is this a problem? How does it impact on well being and functional status? For instance, is it resulting in loss of appetite, loss of attention to personal appearance and hygiene? Does it interfere with activities of daily living? Does it act as a barrier, creating avoidance by others?*	**Comments**	*This statement gives you something to focus on. You can use the manner in which she demonstrates the depression as a vehicle to gauge improvement in the depression.* *Remember: The problem statement is the impact or result of the issue reflected here and now.* *Once you become accustomed to thinking in this manner you will easily develop a more proactive and focused care plan.*
Goal	Will make one positive self-statement/day	**Goal**	Resident will show interest in her personal appearance as evidenced by tending to grooming needs daily and asking for feedback on her appearance from the staff.
Comments	*How does this improve the outcome? How are you going to determine this? What do you want this to result in?*	**Comments**	*You can see how much easier it is to write doable, measurable goals when you have a focused problem statement.*

Comparison of Care Plan Problem/Goal Statements (cont.)

	NOT GOOD		BETTER
Problem	Agitated during care.	**Problem**	Agitated during care as a result of poor comprehension, creating risk for injury to self or staff, and poor hygiene.
Comments	*So, what is the problem? How is it being demonstrated?* *Why resident is agitated is an assessment problem. With a thorough assessment, care planning may end up being a simple set of interventions that will prevent or minimize the behavior problem.* *What is the result or impact of agitation during care? Risk for poor hygiene, risk for injury to self or others; escalation of behavior requiring more invasive interventions such as drugs or restraints to control agitation? Do staff members dread caring for the person, or does the person feel disliked?* *Always determine what is the impact on the resident and the environment. Use four-quadrant thinking (physical, mental, social, and emotional) to ensure a holistic approach.*	**Comments**	*The impact on the person and the environment are the here and now care planning needs.* *The cause of the agitation and indicating what it creates as part of the problem statement facilitates your ability to develop goal statements and create appropriate interventions.*
Goal	Will not be agitated during care or will only be agitated once/day.	**Goal**	Agitation will be manageable as evidenced by neat and clean appearance each day; will not injure self or others.
Comments	*Does this really require comment? Is it doable? Is it appropriate? Aren't there valid reasons a person could become agitated? What does being agitated only once a day accomplish other than a number that says, "See, it's measurable"! The question is, just what are you measuring?*	**Comments**	*When writing goal statements you also need to consider the correctability of the problem. Sometimes problems can't be fixed! The question becomes, what is the best outcome you can hope to achieve?*

Comparison of care plan problem/goal statements: Creating problems where none exists

Not infrequently, we "make up" problems because we think we have to have one when we don't! This is a hangover from regulations of years past, which mandated each discipline MUST have a care plan. As a result, we wrote care plans for EVERYTHING (even though only the surveyors used them!). It was actually a training session to condition us to the idea that care plans needed to be done! Today the regulations require care planning be done as indicated based on a comprehensive assessment of the resident's status. Today's requirements stress care planning based on a holistic care model, not a medical model.

Activities are a good example of creating problems where none exists. More often than not, activities is a supportive intervention rather than a problem or need. How often have you written a care plan like this?

Problem statement	Does not participate in activities.
Comments	*So what? Why is this problem? Whose problem is it—the resident's or the activities department feeling pressed to develop a plan? Why is there no participation? Is it a lifestyle/history issue or the result of a current problem?* *This problem statement is vague. It is about yesterday and tomorrow. The first question to ask is: Is this really a problem for the resident? If so, why? The why is the real problem statement.*
Goal	Will participate in activities three times/week.
Comments	*Sure it's measurable, but just what are you measuring? How does this goal impact on the functional status of the resident? You can't possibly know because you have NOT identified the problem!*
Restated example	Depressed, self-isolating, and refuses to participate in activities. By history was always very social and involved.
Goal	Depression will resolve as evidenced by attending and actively participating in activities on a daily basis.
Comments	*As you can see, the problem was depression—the lack of involvement in activities is how the depression is demonstrated! Therefore activities is NOT the problem, but becomes the vehicle to measure the improvement in the depression.*

Determining interventions

Each team member should ask: Is there anything I can offer from my discipline to help with this problem? Do I have ideas for others that may be of use?

Keep interventions cookbook style when at all possible. Lengthy, verbose interventions may not get read or implemented! Don't hang yourself with interventions that look good on paper, but create hardship to implement or validate.

Interventions must reflect the relationship to the problem and goal. This is automatic if you have considered the preceding rules.

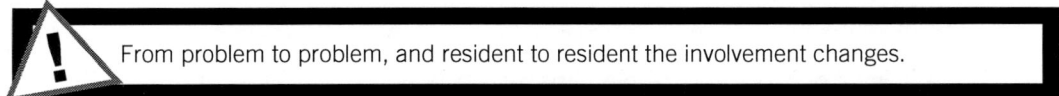

From problem to problem, and resident to resident the involvement changes.

To ensure a comprehensive plan each discipline must reconsider what if anything it can offer to aid in meeting the goal(s). Some require all disciplines to intervene. Others require a combination, and a relative few require only one.

Deciding on accountability

The discipline with the greatest ownership for the problem holds the accountability for plan implementation and modification between scheduled reviews (established target dates). This does not necessarily mean they are responsible for doing the interventions. They are responsible for monitoring and ensuring effectiveness, and alerting the responsible caregiver supervisor if interventions are not being provided as planned and indicated on the care plan.

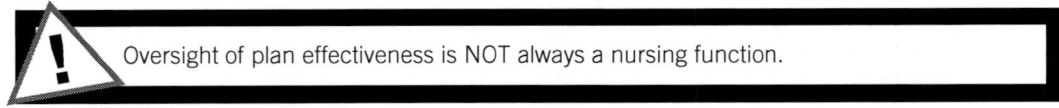

Oversight of plan effectiveness is NOT always a nursing function.

The discipline with the greatest ownership for the problem must take the responsibility to ensure the plan is being properly implemented. The discipline should also be evaluating effectiveness of the plan between team meetings. The frequency of the evaluation will be dependent on the scope, severity, and stability of the problem/need.

Establishing time frames and review dates

These need to be based on the scope, severity, and stability of the particular problem you are dealing with. This is the rationale behind assigning accountability to a particular discipline for reviews that are needed between quarters!

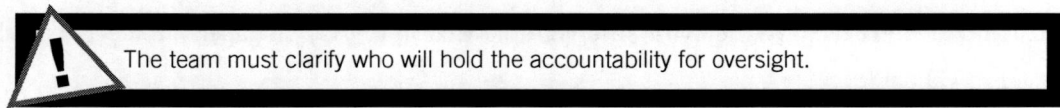

The team must clarify who will hold the accountability for oversight.

Don't assume everyone knows. Consider using the last listed discipline as the vehicle to reflect this.

Oversight does NOT mean day-to-day supervision of implementation. It means periodically checking. If the plan is not being implemented or is implemented incorrectly, the chain of command must be followed to correct the problem. The last thing people need is more bosses!

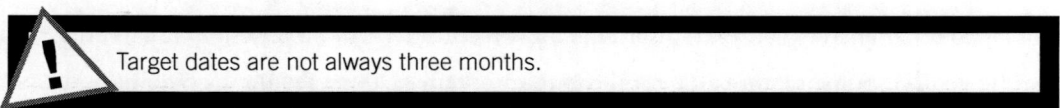

Target dates are not always three months.

Consideration must be given to the scope and severity of the problem. This doesn't necessarily mean that a team meeting must be held for every goal developed outside of three months. It means that the responsible discipline noted above will check the plan on that date, make a note, and take action accordingly.

Before implementing plans, consensus must be sought with resident, family, and those responsible for implementation. Hopefully that will be a formality—if involvement was sought and obtained prior to plan development, a feasible plan will most likely have fallen into place.

Consider the scope, severity, and stability of the identified problems and needs to facilitate priority problem recognition and balanced care plans. This will help to prevent putting the cart before the horse!

We sometimes try to address everything all at once because we are worried if it's not on the plan we will get a deficiency, which sets everybody up for failure.

Placing too much data on the care plan can doom it to failure. Sometimes you cannot deal with one problem until you have solved another. When this is the case, provide a note of explanation as to your thinking and awareness of the problems to avoid problems with surveyors. Use the same scope and severity scale applied by surveyors (when citing deficiencies) to help you prioritize care planning needs and actions, along with your input on the stability of the problem, goal, and/or plan.

Consideration of these three quantifiers will allow you to justify your actions and tailor your plan accordingly!

Scope	Severity	Stability
Pervasiveness of the problem.	**Seriousness of the problem.**	**Current status of the problem.**
Present continuously (3)	Immediate jeopardy to health and safety of self or others (4)	In other words is it shaky or isn't it?
Intermittently but patterned (2)	Harm present or imminent (3)	To what degree is the problem solved and/or what is the likelihood of reoccurrence if
Sporadic (1)	Potential for harm (2)	interventions are withdrawn?
	Minor/of little consequence (1)	

Suggested Integrated Care Plan Format: Components of a Usable and Doable Care Plan

To be used, a care plan has to be people friendly. This means the plan must be accessible to the user, easily read and understood, and kept current. To accomplish these goals the following considerations are suggested.

Component/Area	Primary User	Type of Entries	Initiated by	Reviewed and Updated by	Discontinued by	Location
ADL Care Directives *Provides an overview of mental status and behavior for the caregiver.* *Identifies the particular care needed regarding ADLs.*	Direct caregiver Nursing assistant	Overview of behavior and mental status, strengths, risk factors. ADL performance and staff support including task segmentation, special directions. Particulars direct care needs to know on a day-to-day basis to ensure quality of care and life are maintained and promoted.	RNAC, Unit nurses with assistance of nurse aides Time Frame ❑ On Adm. ❑ Following MDS tracking	Unit nurse and primary caregiver Time Frame ❑ At least monthly ❑ When changes occur	In place over the course of the admission	❑ Binder ❑ Clip-board ❑ Resident room
Immediate/Day-to-Day Care Needs *Predominantly addresses medical, nursing, nutritional concerns that are short term or require focused attention to ensure standards of care are met.* *Content includes acute problems, unstable health conditions/Dx, problems requiring routine monitoring/oversight.*	Licensed nurses Professional staff	Acute conditions Acute illness High-risk problems (e.g., falls, skin, restraint use, new psychoactive med, new continence mgt. program). Chronic unstable Dx Changes in status Skilling services	❑ Licensed nurses ❑ Professional disciplines Time Frame ❑ On adm. ❑ On occurrence	❑ Licensed nurses ❑ RNAC ❑ Supervisor ❑ Other Time Frame ❑ Each tour of duty ❑ As changes occur	❑ Licensed nurses ❑ RNAC ❑ Supervisor ❑ Other	❑ Binder ❑ MAR ❑ Medical Record
Core Plan *Mid- to long-range problems and needs—more quality-of-life-oriented or problems that are well controlled but need ongoing intervention and evaluation to ensure goals are maintained.*	Interdisciplinary Team	RAP/QI-related	Individual team member with IDT consensus and/or IDT as group	Within 7 days of completion of MDS/RAPs Quarterly As needed	Individual team member with IDT consensus and/or IDT as group	Front of Medical Record

ADL Directives

The intention of the ADL care plan is to provide ready access and specific information to the primary caregiver to meet the ADL needs of the resident while enhancing resident self performance and participation where possible.

In order for the ADL directives to be effective, they must be used. Used means accessible and user friendly, with content that provides meaningful, helpful information. This eliminates the practice of keeping them on the chart (too many barriers, too much time to review for the primary caregiver).

Where to keep the ADL directives:

1. In a binder by alphabetical order at the nurse's station.

    *   Advantage: Easy access for updates that may be needed and for nurse review of accuracy and pertinence

    *   Disadvantage: A bit more removed from the primary caregiver

2. In a secure location in the resident's room (be sure it is protected from breaches in confidentiality).

    *   Advantage: On site for caregiver-ready reference

    *   Disadvantage: Possible breaches in confidentiality; less compliance with updates

Author Preference

Binder at nurse's station. Allows the nurse quick access when updates are needed, enhances nurse and aide communication, can be readily reviewed when nurse is evaluating status.

A focused review is recommended to be done by nurse and caregiver at least monthly. Review in conjunction with monthly comprehensive/summary nurse's notes, if used by your facility, is the best action.

NOTE OF CAUTION

Do not keep binder accessible to outsiders, including surveyors! During a survey these need to be pulled and placed with the other components of the care plan. Failing to do this creates a false impression that your care plan is fragmented because it is not physically located with all components together. Record reviews are a tedious process and you will want to make it as easy and convenient for the surveyor/reviewer as possible. Nonetheless, on a day-to-day to basis, keep it accessible to the people who have to use it.

ADL Directives

Name _____ Date Initiated _____

> **Purpose:** To provide direct care staff with individualized information to meet the day-to-day care needs of the resident.
>
> **Direction:** Check all that apply. Use MDS to assist. List interventions staff is to use in meeting day-to-day care needs.

Mental Status and Decision-Making

❏ Recalls day to day   ❏ Recalls past life experiences   ❏ Status varies throughout day   ❏ Knows season   ❏ Knows location of room

❏ Recognize staff names/faces   ❏ None of these   ❏ Decisions consistent/reasonable

❏ Poor (i.e.): _____

❏ Never makes

_____

_____

_____

Communication, Hearing, Vision

Understands: ❏ Always   ❏ Usually   ❏ Sometimes   ❏ Never

Understood: ❏ Always/usually   ❏ Occasionally   ❏ Never

Speech: ❏ No speech   ❏ Clear   ❏ Unclear (i.e.) _____

Hearing: ❏ No problem   ❏ Some difficulty   ❏ Absence useful hearing

Hearing aid: ❏ No ❏ Yes Left Right

Vision: ❏ Able to see   ❏ Wears glasses   ❏ Needs to put on/take off   ❏ Not able to see   ❏ Artificial eye L R

Interventions Needed:

_____

_____

_____

Mood and Behavior

❏ Mood generally good   ❏ Mood is often sad/unhappy (i.e.) _____

❏ Behavior generally reasonable   ❏ Behavior is often problematic (i.e.) _____

Suggested manner of approach:

_____

_____

_____

Special Considerations

Prefers to be called _____

Needs/wants from staff (note particular preferences or things that make resident feel better, enjoy talking about, etc.):

_____

_____

_____

ADL Directives (cont.)

❏ **Fall-Risk Precautions:** ❏ Bed alarm ❏ Chair alarm ❏ Other _____

❏ **SKIN-Risk Precautions:** _____

❏ **PHYSICAL RESTRAINT:** ❏ Belt ❏ Jacket ❏ G/C ❏ Lap buddy ❏ Wrist ❏ Mitt ❏ Merry walker ❏ Side rails

❏ Other _____

Time period for use _____ Circumstances of use _____

YOU MUST CHECK EVERY 15-30 MINUTES AND EXERCISE EVERY 1 –2 HOURS PER POC

Resident Self Performance   Code based on AVERAGE performance   NA = Not applicable/not done

I = Independent, no help or occasional support   **S** = Supervision, oversight, encouragement, cueing   **LA** = Limited assist, resident very involved

EA = Extensive assist, resident does some, staff does most   **T** = Does nothing for Self

Staff Support Codes   Code based ON AVERAGE support   NA = Not applicable/not done

0 = No setup or physical help   **1** = Setup help only   **2** = One-person physical assist   **3** = Two + person physical assist

Resident Performance	Staff Support	Special Instructions, Task Segmentation Needed, Comments, Clarifications Indicate type of supervision and what type of assist needed if LA or EA.
Bed Mobility ❏ Side rails for mobility		**Restorative Nursing Program** ❏ No ❏ Yes _____ **APPLIANCES/DEVICES:** ❏ Ted Hose ❏ Splint Brace _____ ❏ Other _____
Transfer ❏ Bedfast ❏ Lifted ❏ Hoyer ❏ Side rails for transfer		
Walking in Room		
Walking in Hall		
Locomotion on Unit ❏ Cane/Walker ❏ W/C ❏ G/C		
Eating		**Restorative Dining Program:** ❏ Yes ❏ No **Adaptive Equipment:** ❏ Yes ❏ No **Diet** _____ **Supplements** _____
❏ NPO ❏ NG ❏ G-tube ❏ Other _____		

ADL Directives (cont.)

Toilet Use	

Continent Bladder
❑ Yes ❑ No

Catheter
❑ External ❑ Internal

Continent Bowel
❑ Yes ❑ No ❑ Colostomy

❑ **Continence Management Program**

Uses: ❑ bathroom ❑ bedside ❑ commode ❑ urinal ❑ bedpan

Toilet schedule _____ ❑ 1st shift ❑ 2nd shift ❑ 3rd shift

Adult pads ❑ N/A ❑ Always ❑ Day ❑ Night ❑ Outings

Bathing	

❑ Tub ❑ Shower ❑ Bed

Personal Hygiene	

Oral Care	
❑ Own teeth ❑ Dentures ❑ No teeth	

Dressing	

Restorative Nursing Program ❑ No ❑ Yes _____

The Big Book of Care Plans, Second Edition

Immediate Needs Care Plan

Concept and philosophy

Regulations require resident problems and needs to be care planned. The format and method for doing so is an individual facility decision.

The intention of the regulation is to ensure that the care plan identifies the problems and needs and is known and followed. Too often, acute problems are noted after the fact, if at all. Care planning completed after the fact results in a paper-compliant attempt to meet the regulatory requirement. In reality however, it does nothing except take up valuable time in a useless exercise. Outcomes are dependent on caregiver knowledge and use of the care plan. Citations are issued for failing to know and follow the care plan and can result in a deficiency determined to have been avoidable—all because of care plan lack of presence or lack of knowledge and/or lack of use.

To be successful, care plans must be accessible, used, followed, and reviewed. This can only happen when they are readily available, and staff do not have to play seek and find on top of the hectic pace they run during each shift, every day.

Immediate needs care plans (INPOC) are intended to address the problems and needs that require day-to-day intervention, monitoring, or both. If they are buried in the body of a long-term care plan, they are not used. The immediate needs care plan is designed to readily identify and locate resident plans on a day-to-day basis, dramatically increasing the rate of use and compliance.

Advantages of INPOC

1. Ready access for all disciplines. Negates need to go to medical record–enhancing compliance.

2. Easy for supervisor/clinicians to scan for resident problems on the unit, enhancing more timely identification of emerging patterns and trends for the resident or those occurring on a unit level.

3. Encourages timely review of, and appropriateness of actions initiated on new problems.

4. Enhances information for completion of the MDS and RAP review.

5. Encourages and enhances unit nurse involvement and ownership of care plans.

Licensed staff members have little time available for the act of care planning. Often, even the review or completion of necessary supporting documentation is a challenge. When plans and notes are buried in the medical record, the odds for compliance are dramatically reduced. It is next to impossible to oversee compliance, quality of plans, and documentation (which ultimately convert to resident care) when each review requires finding the chart, then opening and digging through it.

People often confuse an integrated, comprehensive care plan with location, as opposed to content and usage. Unfortunately many surveyors have perpetuated this false concept.

Use of the immediate needs care plan component, along with the ADL directives and core plan format constitute the comprehensive plan of care. Use of this concept, coupled with surveyor orientation to the system (on arrival for a survey) can significantly improve your outcomes.

Purpose of the immediate needs care plan

Immediate needs care plans are intended to enhance licensed and professional staff awareness, communication, coordination, and actions regarding the immediate, day-to-day crucial care needs of the resident.

INPOCs are also invaluable in picking up emerging patterns or trends that, if identified, can spawn a different approach to care planning or a further assessment for causative factors. This process begins with where the plans are located.

Where to keep immediate needs care plans

1. In a binder by alphabetical order at the nurse's station.

   - **Advantage:** Ready reference and access for all clinicians. Can be used for report, further facilitating compliance with use and documentation.

   - **Disadvantage:** Another binder to contend with. Potential for outsider access (e.g., surveyor could pick up the book and identify unit issues without any effort (although if you are doing this too, all your issues "should be" addressed and acted on).

2.   With the Medication/Treatment Record.

- **Advantage:** Readily accessible for the nurse; prompts to review and document without additional steps; negates need to go to another source or add another binder.

- **Disadvantage:** Lacks ready accessibility for other team members. You would need to evaluate and anticipate possible difficulties for them, and problem solve.

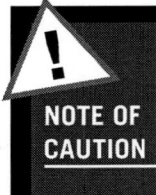

NOTE OF CAUTION

Do not keep binder accessible to outsiders, including surveyors! During a survey INPOCs need to be pulled and coordinated with the ADL Directives and core plan. Failing to do this creates a false impression that your care plan is fragmented because it is not physically located together with the three components. Record reviews are a tedious process and you will want to make it as easy and convenient for the surveyor/reviewer as possible. Nonetheless, on a day-to-day to basis, keep it accessible to the people who need to use it.

Formats

There are several immediate needs formats to choose from, as you will note on the following pages. The choice in formats depends on your facility needs and organizational structure.

The combination of the immediate needs care plan with the nurse's note beginning at the bottom of the page and continuing on the back is designed to keep the writer connected with the problem he or she is documenting. Each plan has its own set of notes. This can be initially confusing, as the staff isn't sure where to document non-related INPOC issues and ends up double documenting (which can be a nice change of pace from no documenting). This problem subsides with use. Another advantage is focused information on a particular problem is all in one place. Therefore, you can readily identify gaps in entries and improve the continuity of the record, as well as easily extract specific data that may be requested on an audit.

A variation of this combination format is the INPOC without nurse's notes on the bottom of the page. You can still start them on the back or you can use a "running" nurse's note that encompasses all nursing notes. With this concept, consider using a problem sheet which identifies which problems are active and which have been resolved. This will facilitate recognition of active plans as well as emerging patterns.

The final variation is a completely different layout. The idea is to readily define each discipline's involvement (if any) with the particular INPOC. This enables the discipline to readily add their "own" interventions. The nurse's notes can be added to the back of the plan, or a running nurse's note with the problem index list can be used.

Content of immediate needs care plan

1. Newly noted areas of risk such as falls, skin, dehydration, etc. If the risk does not materialize after the first quarter, you can consider moving to the core plan section.

2. Out-of-control behavior problems, pain management problems, drug reduction, new problems requiring use of psychoactive medication to correct or control.

3. Unstable health conditions, medications with high risk for side effects, or adverse drug reactions.

4. Wounds, pressure ulcers, acute problems such as falls, new pressure sores, unplanned weight loss or gain, elopements, resident-to-resident abuse, UTIs, URIs, etc.

5. Medicare RUGs (reason for coverage) skilling services.

Immediate Needs Care Plan Problem List

Purpose: This form is used as an index to identify care plan problem/need entries. It is initiated on admission and throughout the resident's stay for short-term, acute, and/or chronic/unstable needs/conditions. As entries are resolved, the care plan is pulled and filed per policy.

MDS Coordinator note: Review the three previous months' entries for patterns and relationships to Core (RAP) Plan problems in conjunction with quarterly reviews.

Directions for use: As plans are initiated note the date, problem, and frequency of charting. On resolution, note the date resolved.

Resident Name _____ Date Admitted/Readmitted _____

Date	Problem	Charting		Date Resolved
		Shift	**Frequency**	
	1	❑ Days ❑ Eves ❑ Nites	❑ QD ❑ QOD ❑ Qwk on _____ ❑ Qmo _____	
	2	❑ Days ❑ Eves ❑ Nites	❑ QD ❑ QOD ❑ Qwk on _____ ❑ Qmo _____	
	3	❑ Days ❑ Eves ❑ Nites	❑ QD ❑ QOD ❑ Qwk on _____ ❑ Qmo _____	
	4	❑ Days ❑ Eves ❑ Nites	❑ QD ❑ QOD ❑ Qwk on _____ ❑ Qmo _____	
	5	❑ Days ❑ Eves ❑ Nites	❑ QD ❑ QOD ❑ Qwk on _____ ❑ Qmo _____	
	6	❑ Days ❑ Eves ❑ Nites	❑ QD ❑ QOD ❑ Qwk on _____ ❑ Qmo _____	
	7	❑ Days ❑ Eves ❑ Nites	❑ QD ❑ QOD ❑ Qwk on _____ ❑ Qmo _____	
	8	❑ Days ❑ Eves ❑ Nites	❑ QD ❑ QOD ❑ Qwk on _____ ❑ Qmo _____	
	9	❑ Days ❑ Eves ❑ Nites	❑ QD ❑ QOD ❑ Qwk on _____ ❑ Qmo _____	
	10	❑ Days ❑ Eves ❑ Nites	❑ QD ❑ QOD ❑ Qwk on _____ ❑ Qmo _____	

Immediate Needs Care Plan

Resident Name _____ Date of Problem _____

PROBLEM/NEED _____
_____
_____

GOAL(S)	INTERVENTIONS/APPROACHES	RESP. DISC.

Target Date _____ Signature/Title of Care Plan Writer _____

❑ Physician notified _____   ❑ Next of Kin notified _____   ❑ Staff informed of plan
                          time   time

Immediate Needs Care Plan (cont.)

Resident Name		Date

PROBLEM/NEED RELATED TO	RESULTING IN	STRENGTHS TO DRAW ON

GOAL(S)	TARGET/REVIEW DATE

INTERVENTIONS	
NURSING	**DIETARY**
	SOCIAL SERVICES
	ACTIVITIES

Immediate Needs Care Plan (cont.)

PROBLEM/NEED _____

_____

_____

GOAL(S)	INTERVENTIONS/APPROACHES	RESP. DISC.

Target Date _____ **Signature/Title of Care Plan Writer** _____

❑ Physician notified _____ ❑ Next of Kin notified _____ ❑ Staff informed of plan
                time   time

Immediate Needs Care Plan (cont.)

NURSE'S NOTES: (Keeping nurse's notes with your immediate needs care plans improves content and timelines of entries. The fewer steps to document, the better the compliance and the easier to oversee.)

DATE	

Nurse's Notes	
DATE	

Immediate Needs Care Plan (cont.)

Nurse's Notes for _____

Directions: You can formulate the information you need in a yes or no format rather than or in addition to narrative nurse's notes. The narrative notes would then be used to explain any no responses or additional information.

	Yes	No	Yes	No	Yes	No	Yes	No	Yes	No	Yes	No	Yes	No	Yes	No
Nurse's Initials																

The Big Book of Care Plans, Second Edition

Core Care Plans

Core plans are the outcome of the completed triggered resident assessment protocols, professional assessments, Quality Indicators, and evaluation of immediate needs care plan content.

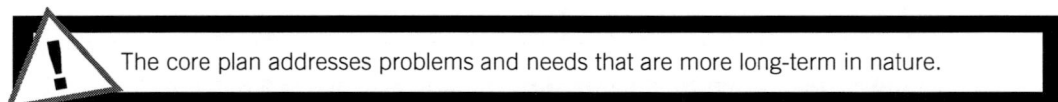

The core plan addresses problems and needs that are more long-term in nature.

Plans are typically more quality-of-life oriented, requiring more staff training to address the particulars for the individual.

Plans also include problems and needs which may require monitoring and intervention, but are well controlled and need only periodic review to ensure the goals and interventions remain appropriate.

These plans are generally overseen by the interdisciplinary team via admission, quarterly, significant-change, and annual reviews done in conjunction with the MDS.

When these reviews are completed it is important that the team critique the other two components of the comprehensive plan to ensure coordination. The ADL directives address the day-to-day needs and staff support required. The immediate needs address the day-to-day high-risk, acute, and chronic medical conditions requiring close scrutiny. As the Interdisciplinary Team reviews the resident with each MDS completion these components of the care plan are also reevaluted.

Deciding where to address the problem or need

Deciding whether to address a problem as an immediate need or a core plan issue is a judgment call. As a general guideline, problems that are unstable, high risk, or require a portion of time to determine their scope or stability are addressed initially as immediate needs.

Not infrequently, when evaluating immediate needs care plans, the team will decide that a problem no longer requires the same intensity of oversight and/or is stable enough that it can be "moved" to the core plan. This might include risk plans where none have materialized over the quarter, or an acute behavior problem that has stabilized, etc.

It is also possible that immediate needs care plans created during a quarter reflect emerging trends that prompt the need for further assessment and creation of a core plan.

Regardless of where you ultimately place the care plan, what is most important is that the plan is known, used, followed, and periodically evaluated for appropriateness and effectiveness.

The professional assessments, care plan, and interdisciplinary team progress notes are essential to support your actions and thinking regarding the care of the resident and the outcomes you will achieve.

Core Care Plan

Name _____

Related RAPs/QI _____

Date Initiated _____

PROBLEM/NEED	GOAL(S) Note target dates	INTERVENTIONS	Resp. Disc.

Signature of care plan writer

Review Dates and Initials

Methods for Creating Immediate Needs and Core RAP Plans

- **Free form or written.** Best used for RAP complexities. Very individualized. Can be written as separate RAP or by combining RAPs. Although the example provided is pretty straightforward, other RAP areas can become a bit complex. It is a good idea to categorize RAPs by indicating the RAP or related RAPs at the top of the care plan page. This makes it easy for the reader to find what he or she is looking for.

> ⚠️ When developing these plans, remember to sort issues from problems. Some RAPs are issues. They aren't going away and are probably creating impact problems in other RAPs (e.g., confused and disoriented [issue] resulting in inability to find bathroom and risk for incontinence; resulting in poor comprehension and risk for combative behavior during care).
>
> See the difference from the "old" way of doing things?

- **Canned.** Typically a problem. The idea is good, but humans have a tendency to put them on the chart without reviewing or tailoring to the individual. The end result is deficiencies and a paper-compliant non-used system.

- **Structured.** A variation and upgrade to the canned format. It encourages individualization while conserving time and providing general guidance and standards of practice. Supervisors can readily identify staff failure to individualize. It is best used for commonly occurring problems that are frequently seen and addressed in a similar manner for all residents and/or have accompanying protocols. Most frequently would be used for immediate needs care planning and restorative nursing services, but on occasion might be located with core plans.

- **Computerized care plans.** Caution must be used for much the same reasons as the canned plans. Failing to tailor ANY care plan format to the individual lends itself to problems. Computers do not take the place of thinking or individualizing resident care needs. Used appropriately, the computer can save time and assist in care plan development.

Sample Free-Form Care Plans

Linked/Related RAP areas: Cognition, mood, nutrition, falls, skin, ADL, PA med

Resident Name: LD   **Date:** 1/6/00

Problem/Need	Goal(s)	Interventions
Severe pain (THE ISSUE), has created escalation in chronic depression and anxiety (THE PROBLEM) resulting in risk for	Pain will be minimized/relieved as evidenced by _____	Follow pain management protocol. Document results in nurse's notes.
P: Reduced mobility	Mobility will not be compromised as evidenced by _____	Refer to ADL Directives, rehab and restorative plans.
Urinary incontinence	Will remain continent of urine.	**Note:** *Avoid duplicating information; always refer to original source site.*
Falls and skin problems	Will be without falls or skin problems.	
Dehydration and weight loss	Weight will remain within 1 to 2# of 125.	Could do referral to ADL directives and reference to structured immediate need plans that would cover these needs.
M: Risk for confusion, disorientation.	Will remain alert and oriented as evidenced by _____	***ADL directives plus SS and AC interventions.***
S/E: Escalation in chronic depression and anxiety creating risk for reduced decision-making and poor motivation to participate in recovery	R will continue to make decisions about care.	Refer to ADL directives.
	R will actively participate in recovery via attending therapy and restorative nursing activities.	List social services and activities interventions to support goal attainment.
	Note: *Goal dates may differ dependent on the scope, severity, and stability of the problems. Determine when is reasonable to revisit the plan—it may well be sooner than 90 days.*	

Interdisciplinary Team Progress Report

Resident Name _____ Date _____

| Type of Review: Medicare Day: ❑ 5 ❑ 14 ❑ 30 ❑ 60 ❑ 90 ❑ OMRA ❑ Admission ❑ Quarterly ❑ Significant Change ❑ Annual ❑ Other |

Quality Indicators that Triggered this Review and Explanation of Relationships/Causes

❑ New Fractures	❑ B&B HR	❑ Fecal Impaction	❑ Dehydration	❑ Psych med HR	❑ Restraints
❑ Falls	❑ B&B LR	❑ UTI	❑ Bedfast	❑ Psych med LR	❑ Little/No Activity
❑ HR Behavior	❑ No Toilet-plan	❑ Weight loss	❑ ADL	❑ Anti-Anxiety	❑ Pressure Ulcer HR
❑ LR Behavior	❑ Catheters	❑ Tube feeding	❑ ROM	❑ Hypnotic	❑ Pressure Ulcer LR
❑ Depression					
❑ NO RX					
❑ 9+meds					
❑ Cognitive					

If admit, significant change, or annual review: Triggered RAPs with Indications for Care Planning

❑ Delirium	❑ ADL/Rehab	❑ Behavior	❑ Nutritional Status	❑ Dental
❑ Cognitive Loss/	❑ Incontinence/Catheter	❑ Restraints	❑ Feeding Tubes	❑ Pressure Ulcer
Dementia	❑ Psychosocial well being	❑ Activities	❑ Dehydration/Fluid Maintenance	❑ Psychotropic Drug Use
❑ Vision	❑ Mood	❑ Falls		
❑ Communication				

Immediate Needs Care Plan Patterns/Trends If Applicable this Review

The Big Book of Care Plans, Second Edition

Interdisciplinary Team Progress Report (cont.)

Directions: Begin by summarizing the resident's status inclusive of Quality Indicators Triggered and clinical relationships of the indicators to each other, if present. If an admission, significant change, or annual review, note the causal relationships of RAPs to each other with indications for care planning.

Include: Summary of Status,   QI Clinical Relationships,   RAP Clinical Relationships

_____
_____
_____
_____
_____
_____
_____
_____
_____
_____
_____
_____
_____
_____
_____
_____
_____
_____
_____
_____
_____
_____
_____
_____
_____
_____
_____
_____
_____
_____
_____
_____
_____
_____
_____

Status of Core Care Plan Goals and Modifications/Additions

Goal codes: **A** = Goal met—discontinue plan   **B** = Goal Met—continue plan for maintenance   **C** = Goal not met—plan revised/adjusted

Problem/Need Area or Plan Number	Goal Status	Rationale for Actions/Plan Changes/Additions (if other than goal met, discontinue plan)

Care Plan, Conference, and Discussion Attended by and Included:

Facility Personnel Signature	Discipline	❏ Resident ❏ Family ❏ Next of kin ❏ Significant other
		❏ Provided input prior to conference.
		❏ Unable to attend, report mailed post-conference.
		❏ Reviewed verbally post-conference with _____
		❏ Resident unable ❏ No interested parties
		❏ Attended, Signature below

Structured Care Plans

It is the user's responsibility to tailor these formats to reflect the needs of the individual. Failure to do so creates risk for deficient practices.

Abrasion/Bruise

❑ IMMEDIATE NEEDS CARE PLAN	❑ CORE CARE PLAN

Abrasion/Bruise

Resident Name	Date

PROBLEM/NEED	CAUSE
❑ Abrasion, site description _____	❑ Side rail ❑ Appliance
	❑ Furniture ❑ W/C G/C
❑ Bruising, site description _____	❑ Self inflicted
	❑ Unknown
	❑ _____

GOAL(S)	TARGET/REVIEW DATE
Will resolve without complication. _____	

INTERVENTIONS

NURSING	DIETARY
❑ Check site and change dressing per order.	
❑ Observe site for infection, inflammation, redness, and tenderness.	
❑ Take extra care during transfer, handling resident.	
❑ Continue interventions on at-risk plan in place.	
❑ Modify at-risk plan in place.	**SOCIAL SERVICES**
❑ Develop at-risk plan.	
❑ _____	
❑ _____	
❑ _____	
❑ _____	
❑ _____	**ACTIVITIES**

Abuse, Resident to Resident

❑ IMMEDIATE NEEDS CARE PLAN	❑ CORE CARE PLAN
Resident-to-Resident Verbal/Physical Abuse	
QI: Problem Behavior Towards Others MDS items: E4b, c A = 1, 2, 3	

Resident Name	Date

PROBLEM/NEED RELATED TO	RESULTING IN	STRENGTHS TO DRAW ON
❑ Verbally abusive when provoked	❑ Risk for harm to self	❑ Behavior is alterable
❑ Physically abusive when provoked	❑ Risk for harm to others	❑ Can be easily redirected
❑ Verbally abusive without apparent cause	❑ Risk for isolation/alienation	❑ _____
❑ Physically abusive without apparent cause	❑ _____	❑ _____
	❑ _____	❑ _____

GOAL(S)	TARGET/REVIEW DATE
❑ Others will not harm resident.	
❑ Resident will not harm others.	
❑ Occurrences will be eliminated and/or resolved w/o negative results.	
❑ Resident will use socially acceptable behavior to resolve conflict.	
❑ _____	
❑ _____	

INTERVENTIONS

NURSING

❑ Monitor resident whereabouts: _____ .
High-risk time or situations include _____ .
❑ Discuss potential triggering events with staff.
Use the following approaches _____
_____
_____
_____
_____
_____

Occurrences
Separate the residents and redirect to: _____

❑ Evaluate for injury or distress and take actions accordingly.
❑ Initiate investigation as to cause/circumstance on EACH occurrence. Document findings in the medical record. Initiate risk management report.
❑ Alert supervisor to occurrence for follow-up investigation and additional interventions.
❑ Discuss occurrence/precipitating factors if known and analyze with staff (and resident, if appropriate).
❑ RN responsible for care. Social services and activities meet next tour of duty to evaluate care plan. Document.

DIETARY

❑ _____
❑ _____

SOCIAL SERVICES

❑ Counseling to vent feelings, explore alternate coping mechanisms.
❑ Discuss with family for suggestions they may have to address the problem.
❑ Ensure follow through on Psychiatry/ Psychology consults.
_____
_____
_____

ACTIVITIES

❑ Use diversional activities to redirect:
_____
_____
_____
_____

Abuse, Resident to Staff

❏ IMMEDIATE NEEDS CARE PLAN	❏ CORE CARE PLAN

Resident-to-Staff Verbal/Physical Abuse
QI: Problem Behavior Towards Others   MDS items: E4b,c A=1,2,3

Resident Name	Date

PROBLEM/NEED RELATED TO	RESULTING IN	STRENGTHS TO DRAW ON
❏ Verbally abusive when directed or care provided ❏ Physically abusive when directed or care provided ❏ Verbally abusive without apparent cause ❏ Physically abusive without apparent cause	❏ Risk for harm to self ❏ Risk for harm to others ❏ Risk for not receiving necessary care/services ❏ _____ ❏ _____	❏ Behavior is alterable ❏ Can be easily redirected ❏ _____ ❏ _____ ❏ _____

GOAL(S)	REVIEW DATE
❏ Resident will not harm self or staff. ❏ Occurrences will be eliminated and/or resolved w/o negative results. ❏ Resident will use socially acceptable behavior to resolve conflict. ❏ Resident will receive necessary care and services. ❏ _____	

INTERVENTIONS

NURSING	DIETARY
❏ Always assess resident demeanor prior to initiating verbal or physical contact. ❏ Gain permission prior to initiating care. If resident agitated cease interaction/activity and return in _____ minutes. Tell resident when you will be back and what you want to do. ❏ Allow control and decision-making as able. ❏ Discuss potential triggering events with staff. See ADL directive for specific approaches to hands on care needs. Use the following approaches_____ _____ _____	❏ _____ ❏ _____

	SOCIAL SERVICES
Occurrences · Separate the residents and redirect to: _____. · Evaluate for injury or distress and take actions accordingly. · Initiate investigation as to cause/circumstance on EACH occurrence. · Document findings in the medical record. · Initiate risk-management report. · Alert supervisor to occurrence for follow-up investigation and additional interventions. · Discuss occurrence/precipitating factors if known and analyze with staff (and resident, if appropriate). · RN responsible for care. Social services and activities meet next tour of duty to evaluate care plan. Document.	❏ Counseling to vent feelings explores alternate coping mechanisms. ❏ Discuss with family for suggestions they may have to address the problem. ❏ Ensure follow through on Psychiatry/Psychology consults. ❏ Contract identifying acceptable behavior and rewards and consequences. _____ _____ _____

ACTIVITIES
❏ Use diversional activities to re-direct:
_____
_____
_____

Accidents/Falls/Injury, At Risk for

❑ IMMEDIATE NEEDS CARE PLAN	❑ CORE CARE PLAN
At Risk for Accidents/Falls/Injury	

Resident Name	Date

PROBLEM/NEED RELATED TO		STRENGTHS TO DRAW ON
❑ Confusion	❑ Wandering	❑ Cooperative, follows direction
❑ Unaware of safety needs	❑ Deconditioning	❑ Recall okay
❑ Vision/hearing problems		❑ Knows limits/risk rehab ability
❑ Poor communication/comprehension		
❑ Gait/balance problems	❑ Paralysis	
❑ Psychoactive drug use	❑ Physical restraint use	
❑ Incontinence	❑ Hypotension	
❑ Desensitized skin	❑ Thin/fragile skin ❑ Careless smoking	

GOAL(S)		TARGET/REVIEW DATE
❑ Free of falls.	❑ Will not burn self.	
❑ Will not sustain serious injury.	❑ Will be free of skin tears.	
❑ PA drugs will be reduced.	❑ Restraint use will be eliminated.	
❑ _____		
❑ _____		

INTERVENTIONS

NURSING	DIETARY
❑ Maintain a clear pathway, free of obstacles.	
❑ Keep furniture in locked position.	
❑ Keep needed items, water, etc, in reach.	**SOCIAL SERVICES**
❑ Avoid repositioning furniture.	
❑ Follow fall protocol.	
❑ Pad rough/sharp edges/side rails.	
❑ Follow toileting plan.	
❑ Provide visual prompts to ask for help.	
❑ Use electronic prompt.	
❑ Refer to Restorative plan.	**ACTIVITIES**
❑ Refer to Restraint POC.	
❑ Refer to Psychoactive Drug/Behavior Management Plan.	
❑ _____	
❑ _____	

Adjustment to Facility

❑ IMMEDIATE NEEDS CARE PLAN	❑ CORE CARE PLAN
Adjustment to Nursing Home	

Resident Name	Date

PROBLEM/NEED RELATED TO	**RESULTING IN**	**STRENGTHS TO DRAW ON**
❑ New to nursing home placement	❑ Withdrawal from normal activities	❑ Able to understand
❑ Recent change in self image	❑ Poor appetite, failure to eat, weight loss	❑ Able to express thoughts
❑ Transfer to new room by request	❑ Social isolation ❑ Resisting care	❑ Strong family support
❑ Transfer to new room: unhappy	❑ Open conflict with others	❑ _____
❑ _____	❑ Wandering	❑ _____
	❑ _____	

GOAL(S)	**TARGET/REVIEW DATE**
❑ Resident will participate in activities and self care as able.	
❑ Resident will be free of signs or symptoms of depression.	
❑ Establish positive relations with others and verbalize satisfaction.	
❑ _____	

INTERVENTIONS

NURSING

❑ Orient resident to new surroundings. Verify understanding.

❑ Monitor appetite and weight and notify dietitian if problems noted.

❑ Monitor for signs and symptoms of depression and alert SS/MD.

❑ Monitor for changes in mood. Notify SS and activities.

❑ Attempt to involve in decision-making and activities of day.

❑ Monitor for attempts to wander, attempt to return to previous room location, any adverse reaction to others. Provide redirection.

❑ Document full assessment in nurse's notes for 72 hours

❑ _____

❑ _____

❑ _____

❑ _____

Notify physician if: Resident not eating/drinking; having weight loss; any adverse reaction to the change in environment; resident attempting to leave or harm self.

DIETARY

❑ Monitor weight: Freq _____.

❑ _____

❑ _____

❑ _____

❑ _____

SOCIAL SERVICES

❑ One-on-one: Freq _____.

❑ Allow to vent feelings, redirect if possible.

❑ _____

❑ _____

❑ _____

ACTIVITIES

❑ Involve in activities of choice.

❑ _____

❑ _____

❑ _____

ADL Decline

☐ IMMEDIATE NEEDS CARE PLAN	☐ CORE CARE PLAN
☐ Decline in ADL ☐ Decline in ROM	

Resident Name	Date

PROBLEM/NEED RELATED TO	RESULTING IN	STRENGTHS TO DRAW ON
☐ New CVA ☐ New Fracture	Decline in:	☐ Motivated to improve
☐ Progressive Dementia	☐ Bed Mobility	☐ Able to follow directions
☐ Progressive Illness _____	☐ Transfer	☐ Understands
☐ Withdrawal from self care/Depression	☐ Eating	☐ Can be understood
☐ _____	☐ Toileting	☐ _____
☐ _____	☐ Bathing/Hygiene	☐ _____

GOAL(S)	REVIEW DATE(S)
☐ Will return to baseline status of _____ .	
☐ Will learn adaptive techniques to permanent change.	
☐ Maintain at current level.	
☐ Slow decline and minimize complications.	
☐ _____	

INTERVENTIONS

NURSING	DIETARY
☐ Discuss need for formal therapy with physician.	
☐ Support resident participation in formal therapy: see related immediate need.	
☐ Refer to restorative nursing program for potential programming.	
☐ Provide pain medication as needed.	
☐ Use aids/supportive devices:	
_____ .	
☐ Provide passive ROM to _____ x/d.	SOCIAL SERVICES
☐ _____	
☐ _____	
☐ _____	
☐ _____	
☐ _____	ACTIVITIES

Anticoagulant Therapy

❑ IMMEDIATE NEEDS CARE PLAN	❑ CORE CARE PLAN
Anticoagulant Therapy	

Resident Name	Date

PROBLEM/NEED RELATED TO	RESULTING IN	STRENGTHS TO DRAW ON
❑ History of embolus	❑ Risk for bleeding	❑ _____
❑ Immobility	❑ _____	❑ _____
❑ History of thrombus	❑ _____	❑ _____
❑ _____	❑ _____	❑ _____

GOAL(S)	TARGET DATE
❑ Will be free of bleeding.	
❑ _____	
❑ _____	

INTERVENTIONS

NURSING

❑ Provide anticoagulant therapy per physician order.
❑ Monitor for bruising
❑ If bleeding noted, contact physician and follow first aid measures to stop bleeding.
❑ Monitor and report lab results to physician.
❑ Use electric razor for shaving.
❑ Avoid bumping and handle gently when hands-on care provided
❑ Monitor BP: Freq _____.

Notify physician if: Lab work abnormal for resident; evidence of increased bruising; evidence of internal bleeding; low BP for resident; uncontrolled bleeding.

DIETARY

SOCIAL SERVICES

ACTIVITIES

Bedfast

☐ IMMEDIATE NEEDS CARE PLAN	☐ CORE CARE PLAN
Bedfast All or Most of the Time	

Resident Name	Date

PROBLEM/NEED RELATED TO	RESULTING IN	STRENGTHS TO DRAW ON
☐ Coma ☐ Self-imposed ☐ Ventilator dependence ☐ _____ ☐ _____	☐ Isolation ☐ Withdrawal from self care ☐ Withdrawal from activities ☐ _____	☐ Activity interests easily adapted to room environment ☐ _____ ☐ _____

GOAL(S)	TARGET/REVIEW DATE
☐ Will be free of signs and symptoms of depression. ☐ Will accept and participate in room activities. ☐ Will accept visitors and staff support. ☐ _____	

INTERVENTIONS

NURSING	DIETARY
☐ Provide necessary support for per ADL directive. ☐ Implement preventative measures for potential skin breakdown: See at-risk for skin breakdown care plan. ☐ Monitor resident for signs of depression: lack of interest in food/fluids, disinterest in eating, sad, pained or worried looks, withdrawal from self care. Notify MD and family. ☐ Reinforce orientation to time and day of week. ☐ Allow opportunities to vent feelings, keep in touch with family/friends. ☐ _____ ☐ _____ ☐ _____ ☐ _____ ☐ _____ ☐ _____ **Notify MD if:** Symptoms of depression persist; resident refusing to eat or drink.	
	SOCIAL SERVICES
	☐ Counseling to allow venting of Feelings: Freq _____. ☐ _____ ☐ _____ ☐ _____
	ACTIVITIES
	☐ Provide one-to-one daily to: _____ ☐ Adapt activity of choice to room: _____ _____

Burns

❑ IMMEDIATE NEEDS CARE PLAN	❑ CORE CARE PLAN
Burns	
CMI: Clinically complex MDS Item: M4b = checked	

Resident Name	Date

PROBLEM/NEED RELATED TO	RESULTING IN	AT RISK FOR	STRENGTHS TO DRAW ON
❑ Radiation	❑ 1st degree burn	❑ Infection	❑ _____
❑ Hot liquid	❑ 2nd degree burn		
❑ Cigarette use	❑ 3rd degree burn		❑ _____
❑ _____	❑ _____		

GOAL(S)	TARGET/REVIEW DATE
❑ Will be free of infection. ❑ Burn will heal without complication.	
❑ _____	

INTERVENTIONS

NURSING	DIETARY
❑ Vital signs: Freq _____.	❑ Monitor Labs: _____ Freq _____.
❑ Wound assessment: note changes in odor, appearance, and drainage.	❑ _____
❑ Pain assessment: intensity, frequency.	❑ _____
❑ Effectiveness of pain medication per MD order.	
❑ Fluid intake and output.	**SOCIAL SERVICES**
❑ Treatment per MD order: _____.	
❑ Provide supervision during smoking.	
❑ Provide supervision with hot liquids.	
❑ Monitor lab work: electrolytes.	
❑ _____	
❑ _____	**ACTIVITIES**
❑ _____	
❑ _____	
Notify physician if: Wound displays symptoms of infection; non-healing wound; persistent complaints of pain with pain medication.	

Catheter, Indwelling

❑ IMMEDIATE NEEDS CARE PLAN	❑ CORE CARE PLAN
Indwelling Catheter	

Resident Name	Date

PROBLEM/NEED RELATED TO	RESULTING IN/RISK FOR	STRENGTHS TO DRAW ON
❑ Neurogenic/atonic bladder	❑ Chronic UTI ❑ Acute UTI	❑ Alert and able to communicate
❑ Poor fluid/food intake	❑ Discomfort, pain	❑ _____
❑ Terminal condition	❑ Septicemia	❑ _____
❑ Pressure ulcer(s)	❑ Embarrassment, curtailment of usual	❑ _____
❑ Debilitating illness:	activities	❑ _____
_____	❑ _____	❑ _____

GOAL(S)	REVIEW DATE
❑ Pain, discomfort will be controlled as noted by _____ .	
❑ Risk for septicemia will be minimized/prevented via prompt recognition and treatment of symptoms of UTI.	
❑ Will maintain usual activities.	
❑ _____	

INTERVENTIONS

NURSING	DIETARY
❑ Provide additional fluids between meals and at bedtime.	❑ Give juices high in Vit C, such as cranberry.
❑ Handle catheter with care, keep below level of bladder.	
❑ Note if meds given for pain management are effective. Discuss modification with physician if indicated.	
❑ Provide catheter care per policy.	
❑ Monitor daily color, odor, consistency, if sediment is present.	**SOCIAL SERVICES**
❑ Be alert for fever, chills, monitor temperature: Freq _____	
❑ _____	
❑ _____	
❑ _____	**ACTIVITIES**

Chemotherapy

❑ IMMEDIATE NEEDS CARE PLAN	❑ CORE CARE PLAN
Chemotherapy	
CMI: Clinically Complex	**MDS Item: P1a = checked last 14 days**

Resident Name	Date

PROBLEM/NEED RELATED TO	RESULTING IN/RISK FOR	STRENGTHS TO DRAW ON
❑ Cancer of: _____ _____ ❑ _____	❑ Oral chemotherapy ❑ IV chemotherapy ❑ Nausea/vomiting ❑ Dehydration ❑ Fatigue ❑ Fever ❑ Infection ❑ Pain/discomfort ❑ _____	❑ _____ ❑ _____

GOAL(S)	TARGET/REVIEW DATE
❑ Side effects will be minimized as evidenced by no emesis, fever, uncontrolled infection, or dehydration. ❑ Will be adequately hydrated as evidenced by _____. ❑ Pain/discomfort will be controlled as evidenced by _____. ❑ _____	

INTERVENTIONS

NURSING

❑ Monitor vital signs: Freq _____.
❑ Assess for complications of treatment: fatigue, nausea, vomiting, pain.
❑ Medicate for comfort: observe non-verbal and verbal expressions/behaviors for potential need.
❑ Assess pain intensity, frequency, and medicate as ordered.
❑ Fluid intake and output: allow resident to choose what to eat and drink.
❑ Avoid spicy, greasy foods post-chemo.
❑ Provide antiemetic per MD order.
❑ IV fluids for hydration per MD order: See IV POC.
❑ Monitor lab work: White count, platelets, HG and HCT per orders.
❑ Be alert for symptoms of dehydration: dry mouth, tenting of skin.
❑ _____
❑ _____
❑ _____
❑ _____

Notify physician if: Persistent complaints/evidence of nausea and vomiting; persistent complaints of pain with pain medication; abnormal lab results; persistent fever.

DIETARY

❑ Monitor labs: _____ Freq _____.
❑ Provide diet per resident request.
❑ _____
❑ _____

SOCIAL SERVICES

❑ Allow resident to vent feelings.
❑ Assist resident and family in coping skills: consult hospice as indicated.

ACTIVITIES

Coma

❑ IMMEDIATE NEEDS CARE PLAN	❑ CORE CARE PLAN
Coma: Not Awake, Totally Dependent on ADL	
CMI: Clinically complex MDS Item: B1 = 1, N1d = checked and G1a–jA = 4 or 8	

Resident Name	Date

PROBLEM/NEED RELATED TO	RESULTING IN/RISK FOR	STRENGTHS TO DRAW ON
❑ Diabetes ❑ Head trauma ❑ Cerebrovascular accident ❑ Unknown ❑ _____	Dependence for all ADL, food, and fluids ❑ Chronic temperature elevation ❑ Aspiration ❑ Constipation ❑ Skin breakdown ❑ Contractures ❑ _____	❑ _____ ❑ _____

GOAL(S)	TARGET/REVIEW DATE
❑ Will present as clean and well groomed. ❑ Will remain adequately nourished and hydrated as evidenced by _____ . ❑ Will be free of skin breakdown. ❑ Will be free from aspiration. ❑ Will have BM at least every third day. ❑ Contracture will not worsen. ❑ Contractures will not develop.	

INTERVENTIONS

NURSING	DIETARY
Refer to ADL Directives for care needs and specifics. ❑ Skin condition check with each bath. Interventions per skin POC. ❑ Lung sounds: Freq _____ . ❑ Bowel sounds: Freq _____ . ❑ Follow bowel regimen protocol. ❑ Provide fluid and food per tube as ordered. See Tube Feed POC. ❑ Provide IV fluids and medication per MD order: See IV and IV med POC. ❑ Provide restorative ROM: See Restorative Care Plan. ❑ Keep HOB elevated _____ degrees. ❑ Suction resident as needed: See suctioning POC. ❑ Monitor lab work: Blood sugars, intake and output as ordered. ❑ Provide medication per MD orders. ❑ _____ ❑ _____ ❑ _____	❑ Nursing to alert dietary of any problems with tube feed. ❑ Weight assessment: Freq _____ . ❑ Monitor Labs: _____ Freq _____ . ❑ _____ ❑ _____
	SOCIAL SERVICES
Notify physician if: Fever develops/persist above _____ ; vital signs diminish; output decreases; complications occur.	**ACTIVITIES**

Congestive Heart Failure

❏ IMMEDIATE NEEDS CARE PLAN	❏ CORE CARE PLAN
Congestive Heart Failure	

Resident Name	Date

PROBLEM/NEED RELATED TO	RESULTING IN	STRENGTHS TO DRAW ON
❏ ASHD ❏ Valvular Disease ❏ Post MI ❏ Arrythmias ❏ HTN ❏ Cardiomoypathy ❏ _____	❏ Fatigue ❏ Dyspnea on exertion ❏ Edema, weight gain ❏ Decline in ADL ❏ _____	❏ Able to communicate needs ❏ Able to perform tasks but is slow ❏ Wants to do more for self ❏ _____

GOAL(S)	TARGET/REVIEW DATE
❏ Lungs will be clear without complaints of shortness of breath on exertion ❏ Will be free of edema ❏ Will participate in ADL by _____ ❏ _____	

INTERVENTIONS

NURSING

❏ Keep HOB elevated _____ degrees.
❏ Assess lung fields: Freq _____.
❏ Monitor Vital signs: Freq _____.
❏ Provide oxygen per _____ at _____ liters per minute.
❏ Provide medications as per MAR.
❏ Break tasks up into small parts with rest periods in between
_____.
❏ Allow resident rest periods throughout the day Specify:
_____.
❏ Teach resident to conserve energy by: _____.
❏ _____
❏ _____

Notify MD if: Shortness of breath persists; vital signs unstable; lung fields with signs of continued congestion; edema persists or worsens.

DIETARY

❏ Na+ restricted diet:
_____.
❏ Monitor weights: Freq _____.
❏ Diet supplement: _____.
❏ Fluid restriction: _____cc Meals:
_____cc Medication _____cc Nursing
❏ _____

SOCIAL SERVICES

ACTIVITIES

❏ Involve in structured activities as able:
_____
❏ Provide divisional activity:
Type: _____
_____
Freq _____.
Instruction for nursing staff:

Constipation/Impaction

❑ IMMEDIATE NEEDS CARE PLAN	❑ CORE CARE PLAN
RISK FOR ❑ Constipation ❑ Impaction	

Resident Name	Date

PROBLEM/NEED RELATED TO	RESULTING IN RISK FOR	STRENGTHS TO DRAW ON
❑ Immobility	❑ Nausea, vomiting	❑ Alert and able to communicate
❑ Poor fluid/food intake	❑ Discomfort, pain	❑ _____
❑ Medication: _____	❑ Loss of appetite	❑ _____
❑ Disease process:	❑ Inability to evacuate bowel	❑ _____
_____	independently	❑ _____
❑ _____	❑ _____	❑ _____

GOAL(S)	TARGET/REVIEW DATE
❑ Will have soft formed bowel movement every two to three days.	
❑ Stool will be manually removed every _____ days.	
❑ Will be free of signs and symptoms of constipation or impaction.	
❑ Constipation will be managed; impaction will not develop.	

INTERVENTIONS

NURSING	DIETARY
❑ Provide additional fluids between meals and at bedtime.	
❑ Encourage movement every few hours while awake if not contraindicated.	
❑ Alert dietitian if consumption is poor more than 48 hours.	
❑ Follow dietary recommendations. Alert dietitian if ineffective or non-compliant with recommendation.	
❑ Note if meds given for management are effective. Discuss modification with physician if indicated.	
❑ Follow schedule on delivery record for checking and removal of stool. Note results and any distress to resident.	**SOCIAL SERVICES**
Specify Bowel Regimen	
❑ _____	
❑ _____	**ACTIVITIES**
❑ _____	
❑ _____	

Dehydration

❑ IMMEDIATE NEEDS CARE PLAN	❑ CORE CARE PLAN
Dehydration ❑ **Actual** ❑ **At Risk For**	
CMI: Clinically complex, MDS Item: J1c = Check; If fever, CMI Special Care, MDS Item: J1c and J1h = Checked	

Resident Name	Date

PROBLEM/NEED RELATED TO	RESULTING IN/RISK FOR	STRENGTHS TO DRAW ON
❑ Nausea/Vomiting	❑ Output exceeding intake	❑ Able to communicate needs
❑ Diarrhea	❑ Poor skin turgor, dry mucous membranes	❑ Able to follow directions
❑ Unaware of need to drink	❑ Fever	❑ _____
❑ Fluid restriction	❑ Risk for constipation	❑ _____
❑ Diuretic therapy	❑ Risk for UTI	
❑ Fear of incontinence	❑ Change in mental status	
❑ Depression	❑ _____	
❑ Resists drinking		
❑ _____		

GOAL(S)	TARGET/REVIEW DATE
❑ Will drink a minimum of 1500 – 2000 cc each 24-hour period.	
❑ Free of symptoms of dehydration: moist mucous membranes, good skin turgor.	
❑ Fever will resolve ❑ Will have a normal BM at least every third day.	
❑ Will be free of UTI. ❑ Behavior will return to baseline.	
❑ _____	

INTERVENTIONS

NURSING	DIETARY
❑ Fluid intake and output daily.	❑ Nursing to alert if fluid intake compromised.
❑ Assess dehydration: tenting skin, dry mouth, cracked lips, dizziness on sitting/standing, fever, increased pulse, thirst, weakness, weight loss.	❑ Provide supplements as ordered: _____
❑ Lab work: BUN creatinine.	❑ Check lab: _____ Freq _____.
❑ Instruct resident and family of importance of fluid intake.	❑ Evaluate weights: Freq _____.
❑ Provide fluid of choice: Freq _____.	❑ _____
Fluid volume recommended: _____ cc qd.	**SOCIAL SERVICES**
❑ Assess urine output for symptoms of dehydration: concentrated urine, strong odor.	
❑ Assess bowel sounds and frequency of BM: provide medication per order.	
❑ Refer Restorative Dining Program: Focus on fluid intake.	
❑ Refer to POC for _____.	
❑ _____	
❑ _____	
❑ _____	
	ACTIVITIES
Notify physician if: Persistent symptoms of diarrhea, nausea/vomiting unresolved past 48 hours; persistent output exceeding intake past 48 hours; abnormal lab.	

Diabetes

☐ IMMEDIATE NEEDS CARE PLAN	☐ CORE CARE PLAN

Diabetes: Injections seven days and MD order change two days or more last seven days
CMI: Clinically complex MDS Item: I1a = Check and O3=7 and P8 =/> 2

Resident Name	Date

PROBLEM/NEED RELATED TO	RESULTING IN	STRENGTHS TO DRAW ON
☐ Brittle Diabetic ☐ Diabetes Mellitus ☐ _____	☐ Need for daily insulin ☐ Need for sliding scale insulin ☐ Risk for hypo-/hyperglycemia ☐ _____	☐ Able to communicate needs ☐ Able to follow directions ☐ _____

GOAL(S)	TARGET/REVIEW DATE
☐ Will be free of signs and symptoms of hypoglycemia. ☐ Will be free of signs and symptoms of hyperglycemia. ☐ _____	

INTERVENTIONS

NURSING	DIETARY
☐ Fluid intake and output daily, and weight daily. ☐ Vital signs: Freq _____. ☐ Fingerstick blood sugars: Freq _____. ☐ Lab work: electrolytes, BUN, creatinine, HG and HCT Fasting blood glucose per MD order. ☐ Be alert to signs of Hypoglycemia: diaphoresis, dizziness, headache, hunger, irritability, confusion, paleness, increased pulse, shallow respirations, restlessness, stupor/semi-conscious. Immediately check blood sugar: Give juice with sugar and recheck blood sugar in 10 minutes. If unable to drink, give instant glucogon and reassess blood sugar in 10 minutes. ☐ Be alert to signs of hyperglycemia: flushed, dry skin, drowsiness, nausea/vomiting, abdominal pain, soft sunken eyeballs, red lips, decreased BP, acetone breath, increased respirations. Check blood sugar: Provide sliding scale insulin if ordered. ☐ Monitor for signs of infection: fever, generalized malaise, complaints of abdominal pain, chills. ☐ _____ ☐ _____ ☐ _____ **Notify physician if:** Persistent symptoms of hypo-/hyperglycemia; symptoms of infection; food/fluid intake changes.	☐ Nursing to alert if change in food/fluid intake. ☐ Provide supplements as ordered: _____. ☐ Check lab: _____ Freq _____. ☐ Evaluate weights: Freq _____. ☐ _____ **SOCIAL SERVICES** **ACTIVITIES**

Dialysis

□ IMMEDIATE NEEDS CARE PLAN	□ CORE CARE PLAN
Dialysis	
CMI: Clinically Complex MDS Item: P1b = check	

Resident Name	Date

PROBLEM/NEED RELATED TO	RESULTING IN/RISK FOR	STRENGTHS TO DRAW ON
□ Renal failure □ Diabetes Mellitus □ _____ □ _____	□ Electrolyte imbalance □ Unwanted weight gain □ Need for hemodialysis □ Need for peritoneal dialysis □ _____	□ Able to communicate needs □ Able to follow instruction □ _____ □ _____ □ _____

GOAL(S)	TARGET REVIEW DATE
□ Weight will stabilize between _____ lbs. and _____ lbs. □ Will tolerate dialysis without complication. □ _____	

INTERVENTIONS

NURSING	DIETARY
□ Monitor fluid intake and output and weight daily. □ Monitor vital signs: Freq _____. □ Follow fluid restriction: Fluids per tray: _____ ccs Fluids with medication _____ ccs. Fluids bt. meals _____ ccs. □ Lab work: electrolytes, BUN, creatinine, HG and HCT as ordered. □ If hemodialysis: Monitor shunt for presence of bruit, redness or swelling at site. □ If bleed from shunt: immediately apply pressure and notify the MD. □ If peritoneal dialysis: Monitor site for signs of infection. □ Utilize sterile technique for accessing the port and de-accessing the port. □ Monitor for signs of infection: fever, generalized malaise, complaints of abdominal pain, chills. □ _____ □ _____ □ _____ □ _____	□ Nursing to alert about weight increases. □ Provide diet/supplements as ordered: _____. □ Evaluate weights: Freq _____. □ Check lab: _____ Freq _____. □ _____
	SOCIAL SERVICES
Notify physician if: Shunt problems: no bruit, bleed; Port problems: symptoms of infection; abnormal lab; persistent symptoms of fluid retention. Signs of fluid retention: peripheral edema, weight gain, neck vein distention, orthopnea, elevated BP, tachycardia and tachypnea.	
	ACTIVITIES

Discharge Plan

☐ IMMEDIATE NEEDS CARE PLAN	☐ CORE CARE PLAN
Discharge Plan	

Resident Name	Date

PROBLEM/NEED RELATED TO	RESULTING IN	STRENGTHS TO DRAW ON
☐ Discharge potential within 30 days ☐ Discharge potential within 90 days ☐ Discharge potential uncertain	Need for training to return to community in: ☐ Med administration ☐ Shopping ☐ Transportation ☐ Housework ☐ Wound mgt. ☐ Money mgt. ☐ ADL activities ☐ Need for support services in the home.	☐ Able to communicate needs ☐ Able to make decisions ☐ Motivated to return home ☐ Support available to return to home ☐ _____

GOAL(S)	TARGET DATE
☐ Will return home with satisfactory return demonstration of care needs. ☐ Will return home with appropriate support services. ☐ _____	

INTERVENTIONS

NURSING

☐ Instruct on medications needs and times, safety, etc.
- Schedule practice sessions: Freq _____
- Discuss medication needs and arrangements for prescriptions and follow-up care with physician.
- Provide written instruction sheet at discharge.

☐ Instruct on wound-care needs.
- Schedule practice sessions: Freq _____
- Discuss wound-care needs and arrangements for supplies and follow-up care with physician.
- Provide written instruction sheet at discharge.

☐ Identify teaching needs for ADL in conjunction with therapy plan of care.
Specify: _____
_____
_____
_____
_____

Notify physician if: Resident having difficulty with tasks to be learned; resident will need additional support other than previously discussed; discharge would be detrimental to resident safety.

DIETARY

☐ Special Diet Instruction: Specify:
_____
_____
_____
_____
_____

SOCIAL SERVICES

☐ Work with family to assess home needs.
☐ Arrange home services, specify:
_____
_____
_____

ACTIVITIES

_____
_____
_____
_____
_____

Edema

❏ IMMEDIATE NEEDS CARE PLAN	❏ CORE CARE PLAN
Edema	

Resident Name	Date

PROBLEM/NEED RELATED TO	RESULTING IN	STRENGTHS TO DRAW ON
❏ CHF ❏ Pulmonary disorder ❏ Renal Disease ❏ _____ ❏ _____	❏ Non-pitting edema ❏ Pitting edema ❏ Pulmonary congestion, SOB ❏ _____ ❏ _____	❏ Cooperates with care ❏ Able to communicate needs ❏ _____ ❏ _____

GOAL(S)	TARGET/REVIEW DATE
❏ Edema will subside without complication ❏ _____ ❏ _____	

INTERVENTIONS

NURSING	DIETARY
❏ Elevate extremity to the level or above the level of the heart. ❏ Perform passive ROM on joints in the affected extremity. ❏ Describe if edema is pitting or non-pitting: Apply pressure with fingers, if it is dependent or unilateral, and the severity of the edema by indicating: 0 = none, 1+ = trace, 2+ = moderate, 3+ = deep, and 4+ = very deep. ❏ Inspect skin color for pallor, cyanosis, or mottled discoloration and document. ❏ Assess for capillary refill time by compressing nail beds or surrounding tissue and by observing the return of usual color; if greater than 1-2 seconds then arterial perfusion may be compromised. ❏ Observe skin for any breaks in integrity, or evidence of weeping. ❏ Provide medication as per order. ❏ Monitor labs as ordered, specify: _____ _____ _____ _____ **Notify MD if:** Edema persists; resident presents with open areas or weeping from edematous extremities; changes in amount of edema or evidence of decreased circulation; abnormal lab work.	**SOCIAL SERVICES** **ACTIVITIES**

Elopement Attempts, Poor Decision-Maker

❑ IMMEDIATE NEEDS CARE PLAN	❑ CORE CARE PLAN
Potential for Elopement: Thinking/Decision-Making Poor	

Resident Name	Date

PROBLEM/NEED RELATED TO	RESULTING IN	STRENGTHS TO DRAW ON
❑ Anger over placement ❑ Anger over care received ❑ Problem adjusting to routines ❑ Conflicts with residents/staff ❑ Looking for familiar surroundings ❑ Follows others out of building ❑ Restless/agitated by environment ❑ Unknown	❑ Resident verbalizing desire to leave ❑ Actual attempt to leave	❑ Cooperates with care ❑ Behavior easily altered ❑ _____ ❑ _____

GOAL(S)	TARGET/REVIEW DATE
❑ Resident will be free from harm to self. ❑ _____	

INTERVENTIONS

NURSING

❑ Initiate resident checks: Freq _____.
❑ Initiate wander guard system.
❑ Alert staff to potential for elopement and actions to initiate.
❑ With any attempt, document circumstances, interventions attempted and outcome. Initiate full-house search for resident. Notify Administrator and DON immediately upon missing resident. Initiate missing person policy.
❑ Assess resident for any harm should attempt be made or be successful.
❑ _____
❑ _____
❑ _____
❑ _____

SOCIAL SERVICES

❑ One-on-one to vent feelings, identify concerns, redirect resident.
❑ Assure resident has proper identification including facility phone number and location.
❑ Discuss with family/support person resident's attempts to leave.
❑ _____
❑ _____
❑ _____

ACTIVITIES

❑ Involve in structured activities.
❑ Provide divisional activity:
Type: _____
Freq: _____.
Instruction for nursing staff:

Elopement, Decision-Making Intact

❑ IMMEDIATE NEEDS CARE PLAN	❑ CORE CARE PLAN
Resident Wants to Leave: Thinking/Decision-Making Intact	

Resident Name	Date

PROBLEM/NEED RELATED TO	RESULTING IN	STRENGTHS TO DRAW ON
❑ Anger over placement	❑ Resident verbalizing desire to leave	❑ Able to make decisions
❑ Anger over care received	❑ Actual attempt to leave	❑ Understanding of risks intact
❑ Problem adjusting to routines		❑ _____
❑ Conflicts with residents/staff		❑ _____
❑ Looking for familiar surroundings		
❑ Unknown		

GOAL(S)	TARGET/REVIEW DATE
❑ Resident will be free from harm to self.	
❑ _____	
❑ _____	

INTERVENTIONS

NURSING	SOCIAL SERVICES
❑ Initiate resident checks: Freq _____.	❑ Discuss implications of leaving including facts about the weather and traffic.
❑ Initiate wander guard system.	❑ Discuss/attempt to arrange alternatives that would ensure safety.
❑ Alert all staff of potential for elopement and actions to take should observation take place.	❑ Ensure resident has proper identification including facility phone number and location.
❑ With any attempt, document circumstances, interventions attempted and outcome. Initiate full-house search for resident. Notify Administrator and DON immediately if found missing. Initiate missing person policy.	❑ Notify family/support person of resident's desire to leave.
❑ _____	
❑ _____	
❑ _____	
❑ _____	
❑ _____	
❑ _____	

	ACTIVITIES
	❑ Provide divisional activity
	Type _____.
	Freq: _____.
	Instruction for nursing staff:

Falls

❑ IMMEDIATE NEEDS CARE PLAN	❑ CORE CARE PLAN
Fall	

Resident Name	Date

RESULTING IN	**STRENGTHS TO DRAW ON**
❑ Fall with no apparent injury. ❑ Fall resulting in minor injury to _____. ❑ Fall resulting in serious injury to _____.	

GOAL(S)	**TARGET/REVIEW DATE**
❑ Will resume usual activities without further incident. ❑ Involved areas will resolve without complication. ❑ _____	

INTERVENTIONS

NURSING	DIETARY
❑ Crani-checks x _____ hours. ❑ Vital signs every _____ hours x _____ hours. ❑ Check range of motion daily x _____ hours. ❑ Treatment as ordered. ❑ Continue interventions on the at-risk plan. ❑ Modify the at-risk plan. ❑ Develop an at-risk plan. ❑ _____ ❑ _____ ❑ _____	
	SOCIAL SERVICES
	ACTIVITIES

Fever with Vomiting

❑ IMMEDIATE NEEDS CARE PLAN	❑ CORE CARE PLAN
Fever with Vomiting	
CMI: Special Care MDS Item: J1h and J1o = checked	

Resident Name	Date

PROBLEM/NEED RELATED TO	RESULTING IN	STRENGTHS TO DRAW ON
❑ Acute infection	❑ Temperature above 100 degrees rectal	❑ Able to communicate needs
❑ Flu	❑ Emesis ❑ Weakness	❑ Able to follow directions
❑ Bowel obstruction	❑ Risk for dehydration	❑ _____
❑ Psychogenic	❑ Risk for altered mental status.	❑ _____
❑ Chemotherapy	❑ _____	
❑ Radiation Therapy	❑ _____	
❑ _____		

GOAL(S)	TARGET/REVIEW DATE
❑ Fever and vomiting will resolve without complication.	
❑ Will be free of symptoms of dehydration as evidenced by moist mucous membranes, good skin turgor.	
❑ _____	

INTERVENTIONS

NURSING	DIETARY
❑ Vital signs: Freq _____ .	❑ Nursing to alert if fluid intake compromised.
❑ Fluid intake and output daily.	❑ Provide supplements as ordered:
❑ Record amount, color, frequency of emesis	_____.
❑ Note bowel sounds, frequency of BM, type and amount of BM daily.	❑ Check lab: _____ Freq _____.
❑ Assess for signs of dehydration: tenting skin, dry mouth, cracked lips, dizziness on sitting/standing, fever, increased pulse, thirst, weakness, weight loss.	❑ Evaluate weights: Freq _____.
	❑ _____
❑ Lab work: BUN creatinine electrolytes as ordered.	**SOCIAL SERVICES**
❑ Assess urine output for symptoms of dehydration: concentrated urine, strong odor.	
❑ Provide antipyretic, antiemetic medication per MD orders.	
❑ If related to recent chemotherapy, provide bland, soft foods. Avoid spicy foods.	
❑ Refer to POC for _____	
❑ _____	
❑ _____	**ACTIVITIES**
❑ _____	
Notify physician if: Persistent symptoms of fever, nausea/vomiting unresolved past 48 hours; persistent output exceeding intake past 48 hours; abnormal lab; persistent fever above 100 degrees rectal.	

The Big Book of Care Plans, Second Edition

Foot Lesions with Dressings

❑ IMMEDIATE NEEDS CARE PLAN	❑ CORE CARE PLAN
Foot Lesions with Dressings	
CMI: Clinically Complex MDS Item: M6c and f = check	

Resident Name	Date

PROBLEM/NEED RELATED TO	RESULTING IN	STRENGTHS TO DRAW ON
❑ Corns	❑ Open Lesions	❑ Able to communicate needs
❑ Bunions	❑ _____	❑ Able to follow instruction
❑ Calluses		❑ _____
❑ Hammer Toes		❑ _____
❑ _____		❑ _____

GOAL(S)	TARGET REVIEW DATE
❑ Open lesion will be healed without complication.	
❑ _____	

INTERVENTIONS

NURSING

❑ Monitor vital signs: Freq _____.
❑ Wound status: size of wound, measurements of depth and width, skin color, surrounding skin tissue assessment.
❑ Complaints of pain, effectiveness of pain medication per MD order.
❑ Refer to a Podiatrist.
❑ Apply dressing per MD order: _____.
❑ Note old dressing for any signs of exudate. Assess color and amount if present.
❑ _____
❑ _____
❑ _____

Notify physician if: Evidence of change in or deterioration in status of wound; symptoms of infection; abnormal lab; culture and sensitivity.

DIETARY

❑ Increase protein needs: Provide supplements as ordered to promote healing: _____.
❑ Recommend vitamins for wound healing.
❑ Evaluate weights: Freq _____.
❑ Check lab: _____ Freq _____.
❑ _____
❑ _____

SOCIAL SERVICES

ACTIVITIES

Foot Lesions with Infection

❏ IMMEDIATE NEEDS CARE PLAN	❏ CORE CARE PLAN
Foot Lesions with Infection and Dressings	
CMI: Clinically Complex MDS Item: M6c and f and b = check	

Resident Name	Date

PROBLEM/NEED RELATED TO	RESULTING IN	STRENGTHS TO DRAW ON
❏ Corns	❏ Open Lesions	❏ Able to communicate needs
❏ Bunions	❏ Infection	❏ Able to follow instruction
❏ Calluses	❏ _____	❏ _____
❏ Hammer Toes	❏ _____	❏ _____
❏ _____		❏ _____

GOAL(S)	TARGET REVIEW DATE
❏ Open lesion will be healed without complication.	
❏ Will be free of infection.	
❏ _____	

INTERVENTIONS

NURSING

❏ Monitor vital signs: Freq _____.
❏ Wound status: size of wound, measurements of depth and width, skin color, surrounding skin tissue assessment.
❏ Complaints of pain, effectiveness of pain medication per MD order.
❏ Refer to a Podiatrist.
❏ Apply dressing per MD order: _____.
❏ Note old dressing for any signs of exudate. Assess color and amount if present.
❏ Assess drainage for color, amount, odor present.
❏ Provide antibiotic per MD order.
❏ Provide medication to area per MD order.
❏ _____
❏ _____
❏ _____

Notify physician if: Wound status unchanged for two weeks in a row; evidence of change in or deterioration in status of wound; symptoms of infection; abnormal lab; culture and sensitivity.

DIETARY

❏ Increase protein needs: Provide supplements as ordered to promote healing: _____.
❏ Recommend vitamins for wound healing.
❏ Evaluate weights: Freq _____.
❏ Check lab: _____ Freq _____.
❏ _____
❏ _____

SOCIAL SERVICES

ACTIVITIES

Hemiplegia

❏ IMMEDIATE NEEDS CARE PLAN	❏ CORE CARE PLAN
Hemiplegia	
CMI: Clinically Complex	**MDS Item: I1v =check**

Resident Name	Date

PROBLEM/NEED RELATED TO	RESULTING IN/RISK FOR	STRENGTHS TO DRAW ON
❏ Intracranial bleed ❏ Transient Ischemic Attack ❏ _____ ❏ _____	Weakness/inability to use ❏ left side ❏ right side Swallowing: ❏ Difficulty ❏ Inability Contractures: ❏ Actual ❏ Risk for ❏ Falls ❏ Skin breakdown ❏ Difficulty communicate needs ❏ Weight loss/dehydration ❏ Pain/Discomfort ❏ _____	❏ Able to communicate needs. ❏ Able to follow directions. ❏ _____ ❏ _____

GOAL(S)	TARGET/REVIEW DATE
❏ Will be free from falls. ❏ Will be free from skin breakdown. ❏ Pain/discomfort will be controlled as evidenced by _____. ❏ Will be able to communicate needs via _____. ❏ Will have food and fluid needs met via tube feed. ❏ Will be able to eat _____ %.	

INTERVENTIONS

NURSING	DIETARY
❏ Monitor vital signs: Freq _____ ❏ Neuro checks: Freq _____. ❏ Effectiveness of pain management. ❏ Ensure fluid availability and/or offer frequently during waking hours. ❏ Keep needed items on unaffected side. ❏ Always approach from unaffected side. ❏ Monitor resident status frequently: observe for signs of distress: complaints of headache, flushing. ❏ Refer to ___ PT ___ OT ___ Speech plan. ❏ See POC for ___ Falls ___ Pressure ulcers. ❏ See Restorative plan(s) for _____. ❏ See Tube Feed POC. ❏ _____ ❏ _____ ❏ _____ ❏ _____ **Notify physician if:** Persistent elevated BP; complaints of headache unresolved with medication; changes in neuro checks.	❏ Nursing to alert if change in food/fluid intake. ❏ Provide diet/supplement as ordered: _____. ❏ Evaluate weights: Freq _____. ❏ Check lab: Freq _____. **SOCIAL SERVICES** **ACTIVITIES**

❑ IMMEDIATE NEEDS CARE PLAN
Hospice

Resident Name		Date

PROBLEM/NEED RELATED TO	RESULTING IN	STRENGTHS TO DRAW ON
❑ Cancer	❑ Persistent pain	❑ Able to communicate needs
❑ End-stage disease	❑ Withdrawal from self care	❑ Able to follow directions
❑ _____	❑ Anxiety	❑ Strong family support
❑ _____	❑ Refusing food/fluids	❑ Strong belief in faith
	❑ Fever	❑ _____
	❑ Other _____	❑ _____

GOAL(S)	REVIEW DATE
❑ Pain will be controlled as evidenced by _____ .	
❑ Anxiety will be controlled as evidenced by _____ .	
❑ _____	
❑ _____	

INTERVENTIONS

NURSING	DIETARY
❑ Follow hospice plan of care.	❑ Liberalize diet and fluids offered.
❑ Consult with hospice about resident needs prior to physician contact.	❑ _____
❑ Encourage to verbalize feelings.	❑ _____
❑ Allow rest periods as needed during care activities.	❑ _____
❑ Monitor for comfort needs, acting accordingly.	❑ _____
❑ Evaluate for presence of pain every _____ hours.	
❑ Assess effectiveness of pain medication.	**SOCIAL SERVICES**
❑ _____	❑ Coordinate social/emotional support needs with hospice.
❑ _____	
❑ _____	
❑ _____	
Notify MD if: Condition worsens suddenly; pain persists despite interventions; code status changes; hospice nurse indicates need to change interventions.	**ACTIVITIES**

Hypertension/Hypotension

❑ IMMEDIATE NEEDS CARE PLAN	❑ CORE CARE PLAN
❑ Hypertension ❑ Hypotension	

Resident Name	Date

PROBLEM/NEED RELATED TO	RESULTING IN	STRENGTHS TO DRAW ON
❑ CVA ❑ Renal Disease ❑ Cardiac Disease ❑ _____ ❑ _____	❑ Persistent elevated/fluctuating BP ❑ Headache ❑ Dizziness ❑ Falls ❑ _____ ❑ _____	❑ Able to communicate needs ❑ Able to follow cues, prompts ❑ _____

GOAL(S)	TARGET/REVIEW DATE
❑ Resident will not complain of headaches, dizziness or fatigue. ❑ Resident BP will be maintained between _____ and _____. ❑ Will not sustain fall with injury.	

INTERVENTIONS

NURSING	DIETARY
❑ Monitor BP: Freq_____. ❑ Monitor lab values as ordered. ❑ Monitor for complaints of headache or dizziness Assess BP lying and standing. Compare to baseline. Notify MD if +/– 10 – 20 pts deviation. ❑ Instruct/support to change position slowly. Avoid sudden shifts. ❑ _____ ❑ _____ ❑ _____ ❑ If Fall occurs: see fall care plan and nurse's notes **Notify MD if:** Symptoms of headache or dizziness persist; lab work abnormal; fall occurs.	
	SOCIAL SERVICE
	ACTIVITIES

Internal Bleeding

❑ IMMEDIATE NEEDS CARE PLAN	❑ CORE CARE PLAN

Internal Bleed
CMI: Clinically Complex   MDS Item: J1j = checked

Resident Name	Date

PROBLEM/NEED RELATED TO	RESULTING IN	STRENGTHS TO DRAW ON
❑ Hypertension	❑ Nose bleed	❑ _____
❑ Gastric ulcer	❑ Blood in urine	❑ _____
❑ Trauma	❑ Blood in stool	❑ _____
❑ History of alcoholism	❑ Blood in emesis	
❑ Lower GI	❑ _____	
❑ _____	❑ _____	

GOAL(S)	TARGET REVIEW DATE
❑ Will be free of signs of bleeding.	
❑ _____	

INTERVENTIONS

NURSING	DIETARY
❑ Monitor vital signs: Freq _____.	❑ Provide foods rich in iron.
❑ Symptoms of bleed: weakness, pale color, shortness of breath on exertion, complaints of feeling tired, rapid pulse, rapid respirations, drop in blood pressure.	❑ Check lab: _____ Freq _____.
❑ Evidence of frank bleed: bright red emesis, stool, or urine.	❑ _____
❑ Evidence of old bleed: dark red emesis, urine, stool.	
❑ Evidence of change in level of consciousness.	
❑ If nose bleed, apply pressure to nasal passages.	
❑ Note amount, color, consistency of emesis, stool.	
❑ Provide oxygen as ordered: See Oxygen POC.	
❑ Monitor lab work as ordered: Hg and HCT freq _____.	**SOCIAL SERVICES**
❑ Provide fluid and blood administration per MD order. See IV POC.	
❑ If administering blood products, monitor for reaction; if present, stop blood and report to MD immediately.	
❑ _____	
❑ _____	
❑ _____	
Notify physician if: Symptoms of bleed identified; abnormal lab work; bleeding persists; vital signs diminish.	**ACTIVITIES**

Intravenous Therapy: Continuous

❑ IMMEDIATE NEEDS CARE PLAN	❑ CORE CARE PLAN
Intravenous Therapy: Continuous	
CMI: Extensive Services MDS Item: K5a	

Resident Name	Date

PROBLEM/NEED RELATED TO	RESULTING IN	STRENGTHS TO DRAW ON
❑ Coma	❑ Continuous feed IV fluids	❑ Able to communicate needs
❑ Dehydration	❑ Hyperalimentation and lipid therapy	❑ Able to follow instruction
❑ Malabsorption syndrome	❑ _____	❑ _____
❑ _____	❑ _____	❑ _____
❑ _____	❑ _____	❑ _____

GOAL(S)	TARGET REVIEW DATE
❑ IV site will be/remain free of signs and symptoms of infection, infiltrate.	
❑ Dehydration will resolve without complication.	
❑ Nutrition will be adequate as evidenced by _____.	
❑ _____	

INTERVENTIONS

NURSING

- ❑ Monitor vital signs: Freq _____.
- ❑ Monitor signs of dehydration: poor skin turgor, dry mouth, change in mental status.
- ❑ Evaluate IV site each shift and PRN for redness, swelling, discomfort.
- ❑ Provide infusion control with use of mechanical pump.
- ❑ If central line provide sterile site care.
    Flush line per physician order; If unable to flush easily, DO NOT force or apply pressure. Stop the procedure.
- ❑ Monitor weight: Freq _____.
  Notify dietitian of weight changes +/- _____ lbs.
- ❑ _____
- ❑ _____
- ❑ _____

Notify physician if: Adverse reaction from antibiotic. Stop med, note signs, IV infiltrate and unable to restart; inability to flush central line; peak and trough lab work results; weight changes +/- _____ lbs.

DIETARY

- ❑ Assess total calories received each day, taking action as indicated.
- ❑ Assess total fluid intake/output
  Freq _____.
- ❑ _____
- ❑ _____
- ❑ _____

SOCIAL SERVICES

ACTIVITIES

Intravenous Therapy: Intermittent

<table>
<tr><td colspan="2">❑ IMMEDIATE NEEDS CARE PLAN   ❑ CORE CARE PLAN

Intravenous Therapy: Intermittent Medications
CMI: Extensive Services   MDS Item: P1c</td></tr>
<tr><td>Resident Name</td><td>Date</td></tr>
</table>

PROBLEM/NEED RELATED TO	RESULTING IN	STRENGTHS TO DRAW ON
❑ Acute infection	❑ IV antibiotic therapy	❑ Able to communicate needs
❑ Pneumonia	❑ _____	❑ Able to follow instruction
❑ UTI	❑ _____	❑ _____
❑ Wound	❑ _____	❑ _____
❑ MRSA		
❑ VRE		
❑ _____		

GOAL(S)	TARGET/REVIEW DATE
❑ IV site will be/remain free of signs and symptoms of infection or infiltrate. ❑ Infection will resolve without complications. ❑ _____ ❑ _____	

INTERVENTIONS

NURSING	DIETARY
❑ Monitor vital signs Freq _____. ❑ Give medications as ordered. Monitor for adverse reactions/side effects. ❑ Anticipate and provide PRN meds: cough, pain/discomfort fever, anxiety. ❑ Evaluate IV site each shift and PRN for redness, swelling, discomfort. ❑ Provide infusion control with use of mechanical pump. ❑ If central line, provide sterile site care. Flush line per physician order; If unable to flush easily, DO NOT force or apply pressure. Stop the procedure. ❑ _____ ❑ _____ ❑ _____ ❑ _____ **Notify physician if:** Adverse reaction from antibiotic. Stop med, note signs, IV infiltrate and unable to restart; inability to flush central line; peak and trough lab work results.	
	SOCIAL SERVICES
	ACTIVITIES

Little Activity

❏ IMMEDIATE NEEDS CARE PLAN	❏ CORE CARE PLAN
Little or No Activities	

Resident Name	Date

PROBLEM/NEED RELATED TO	RESULTING IN/RISK FOR	STRENGTHS TO DRAW ON
❏ Medical condition	❏ Boredom	
❏ Depression	❏ Increasing withdrawal, social isolation	
❏ Cognitive status	❏ Overstimulation, behavior problems	
❏ Lifestyle ❏ Refusal	❏ _____	
❏ _____	❏ _____	

GOAL(S)	REVIEW DATE
❏ Will state satisfaction with divisional activities allowed within medical limits.	
❏ Will be socially involved with others as evidenced by _____.	
❏ Will participate in low stimulation activities such as _____ :	
Freq:_____.	
❏ Will attend activities of choice on a _____ basis.	
❏ _____	
❏ _____	

INTERVENTIONS

NURSING	DIETARY
❏ Discuss current events, past life memories during care activities.	
❏ Provide diversional activities such as watch TV, reading, etc.	**SOCIAL SERVICES**
❏ Note and report any non-verbal expressions or indication of being	
	ACTIVITIES

MRSA/VRE

❏ IMMEDIATE NEEDS CARE PLAN	❏ CORE CARE PLAN
❏ **MRSA** ❏ **VRE**	

Resident Name	Date

PROBLEM/NEED RELATED TO	RESULTING IN	STRENGTHS TO DRAW ON
❏ Wound ❏ Urine ❏ Sputum ❏ Blood ❏ _____	❏ Risk for adverse reaction to antibiotics ❏ Isolation precautions ❏ _____ ❏ _____	

GOAL(S)	TARGET/REVIEW DATE
❏ Resident will have no adverse effects from medications. ❏ Infection will be colonized. ❏ _____	

INTERVENTIONS

NURSING	DIETARY
❏ Contact Isolation ❏ Universal Precautions Use: ❏ Gloves ❏ Gown ❏ Mask with direct contact of _____. ❏ Assess for exudates (color, amount, and odor), and document. ❏ Assess vital signs: Freq _____. ❏ Provide antibiotic per order. Monitor for adverse reaction. ❏ Collect culture specimen: Freq _____. ❏ _____ ❏ _____ ❏ _____ ❏ _____ ❏ _____ **Notify MD if:** Fever persists; exudates with signs of continued infection; culture report remains positive; sensitivity report indicates antibiotic resistance.	
	SOCIAL SERVICES
	ACTIVITIES
	❏ Involve in structured activities as able: _____ ❏ Provide divisional activity: Type: _____ _____ Freq: _____ Instruction for nursing staff:

The Big Book of Care Plans, Second Edition

Multiple Sclerosis

☐ IMMEDIATE NEEDS CARE PLAN	☐ CORE CARE PLAN
Multiple Sclerosis	
CMI: Special Care	MDS Item: P1w = check

Resident Name		Date

PROBLEM/NEED RELATED TO	RESULTING IN	RISK FOR	STRENGTHS TO DRAW ON
☐ Hyperactive reflexes ☐ Decreased/absent superficial reflexes ☐ _____ ☐ _____	☐ Fatigue ☐ Sensory impairment: numbness and tingling, weakness in extremities, facial palsy. ☐ _____	☐ Speech deficits ☐ Contractures ☐ Skin breakdown ☐ Bedfastness ☐ Spastic bladder: urinary retention	☐ Able to communicate needs ☐ Able to chew and swallow ☐ Able to maneuver electric wheelchair with straw device ☐ _____

GOAL(S)	TARGET/REVIEW DATE
☐ Will be free from skin breakdown. ☐ Will have no evidence of pain during range of motion. ☐ Will have BM at a min. of every 3rd day per bowel regimen. ☐ Will be able to eat ___ %. ☐ Will be able to communicate needs via: _____. ☐ Will be free of infections. ☐ Will have food and fluid needs met via tube feed.	

INTERVENTIONS

NURSING	DIETARY
☐ Monitor vital signs: Freq_____. ☐ Monitor weight: Freq _____. ☐ Monitor gag reflex: Refer to Speech Therapy. ☐ Verbal and non-verbal communication: Refer to Speech Therapy. ☐ Monitor resident status frequently: observe for signs of distress: urinary or bowel problems. ☐ Provide catheter care. Monitor output shift. Be alert to distention: make sure tubing is not kinked or clogged. Flush per MD order: _____. ☐ See At Risk for Pressure Ulcer POC. ☐ See Restorative POC for _____. ☐ See Tube Feed POC. ☐ Refer to PT/OT. ☐ Avoid isolation potential: transfer to WC, encourage wheelchair activity. ☐ Be alert to numbness: test water temperatures before resident use. ☐ _____ ☐ _____ **Notify physician if:** Deterioration in neurological status; abnormal lab work.	☐ Nursing to alert if change in food/fluid intake ☐ Provide diet/supplements as ordered: _____ ☐ Evaluate weights: Freq _____ ☐ Check lab: _____ Freq _____ **SOCIAL SERVICES** **ACTIVITIES**

Open Lesions with Treatment

❏ IMMEDIATE NEEDS CARE PLAN	❏ CORE CARE PLAN

Open Lesion with Treatment

CMI: Special Care   MDS Item: M4c and M5g and/or H = Checked

Resident Name	Date

PROBLEM/NEED RELATED TO	RESULTING IN	STRENGTHS TO DRAW ON
❏ _____ ❏ _____ ❏ _____	❏ Open lesion location: _____ ❏ _____	❏ Able to communicate needs ❏ Able to follow directions ❏ _____ ❏ _____

GOAL(S)	TARGET/REVIEW DATE
❏ Lesion will be healed without complication. ❏ _____ ❏ _____	

INTERVENTIONS

NURSING

❏ Monitor vital signs: Freq _____.

❏ Wound status: Approximation of wound, assessment of surrounding tissue, presence of staples, sutures where applicable.

❏ Complaints of pain, effectiveness of pain medication per MD order.

❏ Apply medicated ointment per MD order.

❏ Apply dressing per MD order: _____

_____

❏ Note old dressing for any signs of exudate. Assess color and amount if present.

❏ Be alert to any signs of infection: drainage, odor, redness of surrounding tissue, red streaking up the extremity.

❏ Remove sutures/staples per MD order: _____.

_____

❏ Follow up appointment: _____.

❏ Keep Dietary informed of wound status: Freq _____.

❏ _____

❏ _____

❏ _____

Notify physician if: Wound status unchanged for two weeks in a row; evidence of change in or deterioration in status of wound; symptoms of infection.

DIETARY

❏ Increase protein needs: Provide supplements as ordered to promote healing:_____.

❏ Recommend vitamins for wound healing

❏ Check lab: _____ Freq _____.

❏ Evaluate weights: Freq _____.

❏ _____

SOCIAL SERVICES

ACTIVITIES

Oxygen Use

❑ IMMEDIATE NEEDS CARE PLAN	❑ CORE CARE PLAN

Oxygen Use

CMI: Clinically Complex   **MDS Item: P1g = checked**

Resident Name	Date

PROBLEM/NEED RELATED TO	RESULTING IN	STRENGTHS TO DRAW ON
❑ History of COPD	❑ Shortness of breath/anxiety	❑ Able to communicate needs
❑ _____	❑ _____	❑ Able to follow directions
❑ _____	❑ _____	❑ _____
		❑ _____

GOAL(S)	TARGET/REVIEW DATE
❑ Will be able to perform ADL without complaint of shortness of breath.	
❑ _____	

INTERVENTIONS

NURSING

❑ Monitor vital signs: Freq _____.

❑ Lung fields/breath sounds: Freq _____.

❑ Pulse oximetry: Freq _____.

❑ Shortness of breath: assess for pain and discomfort with breathing.

❑ Sputum/increased secretions not cleared by cough.

❑ Provide PRN medications: cough, pain, discomfort, anxiety.

❑ Instruct resident in breathing techniques: purse lip, cough and deep breathing: Freq _____.

❑ Provide oxygen at _____ Liters per min:

____ Intermittent ____ Continuous ____ Mask ____ Nasal cannula.

❑ Prevent irritation/pressure from developing from oxygen tubing by:

_____

❑ Refer to Respiratory Therapy

❑ _____

❑ _____

Notify physician if: Sputum changes in color, amount and consistency; lung field remains diminished or if sounds are absent in any area; increased complaints of difficulty breathing; pulse oximetry less than _____%.

DIETARY

❑ Provide supplements as ordered:

_____.

❑ Check lab: _____ Freq _____.

❑ _____

SOCIAL SERVICES

ACTIVITIES

Pain

❑ IMMEDIATE NEEDS CARE PLAN	❑ CORE CARE PLAN
Pain	

Resident Name	Date

PROBLEM/NEED RELATED TO	RESULTING IN	STRENGTHS TO DRAW ON
❑ Back ❑ Bone ❑ Headache ❑ Chest during usual activities ❑ Hip ❑ Incision ❑ Stomach ❑ Joint other than hip ❑ Soft tissue pain ❑ Other, specify: _____	❑ Complaints of pain less than daily ❑ Complaints of pain daily ❑ Mild pain ❑ Moderate pain ❑ Times when pain is excruciating ❑ Unable to express pain; shows evidence of pain by: _____	❑ Able to communicate needs ❑ Able to express level of pain ❑ _____ ❑ _____ ❑ _____

GOAL(S)	TARGET/REVIEW DATE
❑ Will be free of pain complaints. ❑ Will display signs of comfort, no grimacing or _____ . ❑ Will report pain resolved with pain medication and other interventions. ❑ Will report pain less than daily.	

INTERVENTIONS

NURSING	DIETARY
❑ Assess symptoms of pain on occurrence and document location and pain scale as reported by the resident. ❑ Provide quiet environment. ❑ Offer calming music, TV per resident request. ❑ Offer back rub, warm blankets. ❑ Provide pain medication as prescribed. ❑ Check vital signs: Freq _____ . ❑ _____ ❑ _____ ❑ _____	❑ Offer comfort foods per resident request. ❑ _____ ❑ _____
Notify physician if: Pain persists despite intervention; vital signs are out of normal range along with pain persistence.	**SOCIAL SERVICES** ❑ Provide opportunity to vent feelings ❑ _____ ❑ _____ **ACTIVITIES** ❑ Involve in structured activities as able. ❑ Provide divisional activity: Type: _____ _____ Freq: _____ Instruction for nursing staff:

Pneumonia

❏ IMMEDIATE NEEDS CARE PLAN	❏ CORE CARE PLAN

Pneumonia

❏ **Pneumonia with Fever   CMI: Special Care   MDS Item: 12e and J1h**
❏ **Pneumonia: Respiratory Treatments Seven Days   CMI: Special Care   MDS Item: 12e and 1bdA = 7**

Resident Name	Date

PROBLEM/NEED RELATED TO	RESULTING IN	STRENGTHS TO DRAW ON
❏ History of COPD ❏ Acute infection ❏ _____ ❏ _____	Cough ❏ Non productive ❏ Productive ❏ Shortness of breath ❏ Anxiety ❏ Refusing food/fluids ❏ Fever	❏ Able to communicate needs ❏ Able to follow directions ❏ _____

GOAL(S)	REVIEW DATE
❏ Pneumonia will resolve without complications. ❏ Will resume normal food/fluid intake. ❏ Anxiety will be controlled as evidenced by _____. ❏ _____ ❏ _____	

INTERVENTIONS

NURSING

❏ Monitor vital signs: Freq _____.
❏ Assess breath sounds: Freq _____.
❏ Evaluate shortness of breath for pain/discomfort with breathing; provide meds as ordered.
❏ Suction for sputum/increased secretions not cleared by cough.
❏ Administer antibiotics: monitor for any adverse reaction to drug.
❏ Provide PRN medications; cough, pain, discomfort, anxiety.
❏ Instruct resident in breathing techniques: purse lip, cough, and deep breathing: Freq _____.
❏ Provide oxygen at ____ Liters per min: ____ Intermittent ___ Continuous ___Mask ___ Nasal cannula.
❏ Prevent irritation/pressure from developing from oxygen tubing by:

_____.

❏ Provide respiratory treatments per MD order:
❏ Refer to Respiratory Therapy.
❏ _____
❏ _____

Notify physician if: Any adverse reaction to antibiotic: stop medication, note reaction symptoms; sputum changes in color; lung field remains diminished or if sounds are absent in any area, increased complaints of difficulty breathing, persistent fever.

DIETARY

❏ Instruct nursing to alert to compromised fluid intake.
❏ Assure fluid intake to _____ ccs q hr.
❏ Provide supplement: _____.
❏ Check lab: _____ Freq _____.
❏ _____
❏ _____

SOCIAL SERVICES

ACTIVITIES

Pneumonia, Trach, Suctioning

❑ IMMEDIATE NEEDS CARE PLAN	❑ CORE CARE PLAN
Pneumonia/Tracheotomy/Suctioning	
CMI: Extensive Services MDS Item: 12e, P1I, and P1j	

Resident Name	Date

PROBLEM/NEED RELATED TO	RESULTING IN	STRENGTHS TO DRAW ON
❑ History of COPD	❑ Cough: productive	❑ Able to communicate needs
❑ Acute Infection	❑ Inability to clear secretions, trach suctioning	❑ Able to follow directions
❑ _____	❑ _____	❑ _____
❑ _____		❑ _____

GOAL(S)	TARGET/REVIEW DATE
❑ Trach will be patent, free of occlusions.	
❑ Pneumonia will resolve without complications.	
❑ _____	
❑ _____	

INTERVENTIONS

NURSING	DIETARY
❑ Monitor vital signs: Freq _____.	
❑ Assess lung fields/breath sounds: Freq _____.	
❑ Evaluate shortness of breath for pain/discomfort, anxiety, fluid in lungs.	
❑ Evaluate and document sputum/increased secretions.	
❑ Suction PRN as ordered. Record frequency/number of times each shift.	
❑ Provide trach care as ordered and PRN for increased secretions.	
❑ Minimize irritation of trach site by _____.	
❑ Ventilator settings/MD order.	
❑ Respond promptly to alarm sounding. Evaluate cause and correct. If unable to correct, ambu bag resident, attempt to suction.	**SOCIAL SERVICES**
❑ Give antibiotics as ordered monitoring drug adverse reactions/side effects.	
❑ Give PRN meds as indicated for cough, pain/discomfort, anxiety.	
❑ Allay fears, instruct as to what you are doing, provide reassurance.	
❑ Refer also to Respiratory Therapy plan.	
❑ _____	
❑ _____	
❑ _____	
Notify physician if: Adverse reaction from medications, sputum changes in color, consistency, amount indicating worsening, diminished or absent lung sounds, airway difficulties not relieved by suctioning.	**ACTIVITIES**

Pneumonia with Suctioning

❑ IMMEDIATE NEEDS CARE PLAN	❑ CORE CARE PLAN
Pneumonia with Suctioning	
CMI: Extensive Services MDS Items: I2e, P1i, and P1j	

Resident Name	Date

PROBLEM/NEED RELATED TO	**RESULTING IN**	**STRENGTHS TO DRAW ON**
❑ History of COPD	❑ Cough: non-productive	❑ Able to communicate needs
❑ Acute infection	❑ Cough: productive	❑ Able to follow instruction
❑ _____	❑ Unable clear secretions, suctioning required	❑ _____
❑ _____	❑ Shortness of breath ❑ Anxiety	❑ _____
❑ _____	❑ Tracheotomy	❑ _____
	❑ _____	

GOAL(S)	**TARGET/REVIEW DATE**
❑ Pneumonia will resolve without complication.	
❑ Trach will remain patent, free of occlusion. ❑ Site will be without inflammations.	
❑ Anxiety will be controlled with use of _____.	
❑ _____	

INTERVENTIONS

NURSING	DIETARY
❑ Monitor vital signs: Freq _____.	
❑ Assess lung fields/breath sounds: Freq _____.	
❑ Evaluate shortness of breath for pain/discomfort, anxiety, fluid in lungs.	
❑ Evaluate and document sputum/increased secretions.	
❑ Suction PRN as ordered. Record frequency/number of times each shift.	
❑ Provide trach care as ordered and PRN for increased secretions.	
❑ Minimize irritation of trach site by _____.	
❑ Give antibiotics as ordered monitoring drug adverse reactions/side effects.	**SOCIAL SERVICES**
❑ Give PRN meds as indicated for cough, pain/discomfort, anxiety.	
❑ Allay fears, instruct as to what you are doing, provide reassurance.	
❑ Refer also to Respiratory Therapy plan.	
❑ _____	
❑ _____	
Notify physician if: Adverse reaction from medications, sputum changes in color, consistency, amount indicating worsening, diminished or absent lung sounds, increasing complaints of shortness of breath and escalating/ uncontrolled anxiety.	**ACTIVITIES**

Pressure Ulcers

❏ IMMEDIATE NEEDS CARE PLAN	❏ CORE CARE PLAN

Pressure Ulcer(s)

❏ **Ulcers: 2+ sites over all stages   CMI: Special Care   MDS Item: M2b = > 0 and M5e = Checked**
❏ **Pressure Ulcers: Stages 3 and/or 4   CMI: Special Care   MDS Item: M2b = > 0 and M5e = Checked**

Resident Name	Date

PROBLEM/NEED RELATED TO	RESULTING IN	STRENGTHS TO DRAW ON
❏ Diabetes	Locations	❏ Able to communicate needs
❏ Peripheral Vascular Disease	❏ _____	❏ Able to follow directions
❏ Immobility	❏ _____	❏ _____
❏ Refusal to comply	❏ _____	
❏ _____	❏ _____	

GOAL(S)	TARGET/REVIEW DATE
❏ Ulcers will be healed without complication.	
❏ _____	
❏ _____	

INTERVENTIONS

NURSING

❏ Monitor vital signs: Freq _____.
❏ Wound status: size of wound: measurements of depth and width, skin color, surrounding skin tissue assessment weekly.
❏ Complaints of pain, effectiveness of pain medication per MD order.
❏ Apply medicated ointment per MD order.
❏ Apply dressing per MD order: _____.
❏ Note old dressing for any signs of exudate. Assess color and amount if present.
❏ Be alert to any signs of infection: drainage, odor, redness of surrounding tissue, red streaking up the extremity.
❏ Refer to PT plan of treatment.
❏ Keep Dietary informed of wound status: Freq _____.
❏ _____
❏ _____
❏ _____
❏ _____

Notify physician if: Wound status unchanged for two weeks in a row; evidence of change in or deterioration in status of wound; symptoms of infection.

DIETARY

❏ Increase protein needs: Provide supplements as ordered to promote healing: _____.
❏ Recommend vitamins for wound healing
❏ Check lab: _____ Freq _____
❏ Evaluate weights: Freq _____
❏ _____

SOCIAL SERVICES

ACTIVITIES

Psychoactive Medication

❑ IMMEDIATE NEEDS CARE PLAN	❑ CORE CARE PLAN
Psychoactive Medication ❑ **New admission** ❑ **New order**	

Resident Name	Date

PROBLEM/NEED RELATED TO	RESULTING IN	STRENGTHS TO DRAW ON
❑ New admission, need/impact of med needs to be evaluated. ❑ Behavior problem, not easily altered. ❑ _____	❑ Possible adverse effects ❑ Potential opportunity to discontinue use ❑ New use of med, risk for adverse effects	❑ _____ ❑ _____ ❑ _____ ❑ _____

GOAL(S)	REVIEW DATE
❑ Prompt recognition and intervention if side effects occur. ❑ Need for continuing use of medication will be determined. ❑ _____ ❑ _____	❑ 7 days ❑ 14 days ❑ 21 days ❑ 30 days ❑

INTERVENTIONS

NURSING	DIETARY
❑ Complete side effects monitor per protocol. Take actions if indicated by change in indicators. ❑ Follow non-medical behavior management plan as per care plan. ❑ Monitor mood or behavior change. Meet with SS and activities per protocol to evaluate status. ❑ If nutrition concern, monitor weight: Freq _____. ❑ If hydration concern monitor fluid intake/output: Freq _____. ❑ _____ ❑ _____ ❑ _____ ❑ _____ ❑ _____	Monitor weight and hydration status: Freq _____
	SOCIAL SERVICES ❑ Provide counseling/mood/behavior plan. ❑ Evaluate mood and/or behavior for patterns of improvement or deterioration.
	ACTIVITIES ❑ Provide activities/mood or behavior plan. ❑ Evaluate impact on participation in activities

Quadriplegia

❑ IMMEDIATE NEEDS CARE PLAN	❑ CORE CARE PLAN
Quadriplegia	
CMI: Special Care	**MDS Item: P1z = check**

Resident Name	Date

PROBLEM/NEED RELATED TO	RESULTING IN	RISK FOR	STRENGTHS TO DRAW ON
❑ Trauma ❑ CVA ❑ _____ ❑ _____ ❑ _____	❑ Loss of sweating reflex ❑ Bladder distention and incontinence ❑ Muscular spasms ❑ _____ ❑ _____	❑ Contractures ❑ Constipation ❑ Skin Breakdown ❑ Bedfast all or most of time ❑ Acute medical emergency: autonomic dysreflexia	❑ Able to communicate needs ❑ Able to chew and swallow ❑ Able to maneuver electric wheelchair with straw device ❑ _____

GOAL(S)	TARGET/REVIEW DATE
❑ Will be free from skin breakdown ❑ Will have no evidence of pain during range of motion. ❑ Will have BM min. of every 3rd day/bowel regimen. ❑ Will be able to eat _____ %. ❑ Will be able to communicate needs via: _____. ❑ Will be free of infections. ❑ Will have food and fluid needs met via tube feed.	

INTERVENTIONS

NURSING

❑ Monitor vital signs: Freq _____.
❑ Monitor weight: Freq _____.
❑ Monitor gag reflex: Refer to Speech Therapy.
❑ Verbal and non-verbal communication: Refer to Speech Therapy.
❑ Monitor resident status frequently: observe for signs of distress: complaints of headache, flushing, restlessness. Be alert to possible autonomic dysreflexia. Determine cause and attempt to correct cause (e.g., constipation, bladder distention).
❑ Provide oral hygiene: Freq _____.
❑ Provide catheter care. Monitor output shift. Be alert to distention: make sure tubing is not kinked or clogged. Flush per MD order: _____.
❑ Provide/develop with resident exercise or signals that will help stimulate urge to defecate: digital rectal stimulation: _____.
suppository schedule: _____.
❑ See At Risk for Pressure Ulcer POC.
❑ See Restorative Range for _____.
❑ See Tube Feed POC.
❑ Refer to PT/OT.
❑ Avoid isolation potential: transfer to WC, encourage wheelchair activity.
❑ _____
❑ _____
❑ _____

Notify physician if: Signs of autonomic dysreflexia; abnormal lab work.

DIETARY

❑ Nursing to alert if change in food/fluid intake.
❑ Provide diet/supplements as ordered: _____.
❑ Evaluate weights: Freq _____.
❑ Check lab: _____ Freq _____.

SOCIAL SERVICES

ACTIVITIES

The Big Book of Care Plans, Second Edition

Radiation

□ IMMEDIATE NEEDS CARE PLAN	□ CORE CARE PLAN
CMI: Special Care	**Radiation** **MDS Item: P1h = checked last 14 days**

Resident Name		Date

PROBLEM/NEED RELATED TO	RESULTING IN/RISK FOR	STRENGTHS TO DRAW ON
□ Cancer of: _____ _____ □ _____	Radiation therapy: □ Internal □ External □ Nausea/vomiting □ Fatigue □ Fever □ Infection □ Skin irritation, radiation burn □ Erosion/bleed at implant site □ _____	□ _____ □ _____

GOAL(S)	TARGET/REVIEW DATE
□ Will be free of infection. □ Skin will be free of irritation, burn. □ Side effects will be minimized as evidenced by: no emesis, fever, or symptoms of infection. □ _____ _____	

INTERVENTIONS

NURSING

- □ Monitor skin areas: Freq _____.
- □ Monitor vital signs: Freq _____.
- □ Assessment of side effects: fatigue, nausea, vomiting, pain: Notify MD if unable to control with medication per MD order.
- □ Assessment of site for symptoms of infection: redness, swelling, warm to touch, fever.
- □ Assessment of food and fluid intake: Notify dietary.
- □ Keep skin clean. Avoid using drying lotions.
- □ Maintain radiation markings: do not attempt to wash off.
- □ Provide isolation techniques for internal radiation.
- □ Allow resident to vent feelings and express concerns related to isolation: Refer to activities and social services.
- □ Cover broken areas with dressing, using stretch-type dressing to hold in place, avoid bandages and tape which can irritate skin and cause injury when removed.
- □ _____
- □ _____

Notify physician if: Persistent complaints/evidence of nausea and vomiting; persistent complaints of pain with pain medication; abnormal lab results; persistent fever.

DIETARY

- □ Monitor labs: _____ Freq _____.
- □ Provide diet per resident request. Allow choice.
- □ Monitor weights: Freq _____.
- □ _____

SOCIAL SERVICES

- □ Allow resident to vent feelings.
- □ Assist resident and family in coping skills; consult hospice as indicated.

ACTIVITIES

Rashes

☐ IMMEDIATE NEEDS CARE PLAN	☐ CORE CARE PLAN
Rashes	

Resident Name	Date

PROBLEM/NEED RELATED TO	RESULTING IN	STRENGTHS TO DRAW ON
☐ Adverse reaction to medication ☐ Allergy, specify: _____ ☐ Incontinence ☐ Dry skin ☐ _____	☐ Red, raised, or blotchy patches on skin ☐ Itching ☐ Scratching ☐ _____	☐ Able to communicate needs ☐ Able to be understood ☐ _____ ☐ _____

GOAL(S)	TARGET/REVIEW DATE
☐ Skin will be free of red, raised, or patchy blotches. ☐ Resident will be free of itching and scratching. ☐ _____	

INTERVENTIONS

NURSING	DIETARY
☐ Provide medication per MD order to alleviate itching/scratching. ☐ Assess for cause of rash and attempt to correct the problem: ☐ If related to incontinence products, remove product and attempt a change in toileting plan. See Urinary Incontinence Plan. ☐ If related to medication, stop medication per MD instruction. Indicate possible allergy on medical record. Alert Pharmacy. ☐ If self inflicted, related to anxiety symptoms, notify MD. Provide gloves or protective hand cover to avoid breaking open skin. ☐ Assess for signs of infection. ☐ See ADL directive for special skin care products for bathing. ☐ _____ ☐ _____ ☐ _____ **Notify MD if:** Itching, scratching persists; areas become infected; interventions make no change.	
	SOCIAL SERVICES
	ACTIVITIES

Rehab Therapy

❏ IMMEDIATE NEEDS CARE PLAN	❏ CORE CARE PLAN
Rehab Therapy	

Resident Name		Date

PROBLEM/ NEED RELATED TO	RESULTING IN	STRENGTHS TO DRAW ON
_____	Rehab Therapy for	❏ Motivated to work at program.
_____	❏ OT ❏ PT ❏ Speech	❏ _____
_____	❏ Other _____	❏ _____

GOAL(S)	TARGET/REVIEW DATE
❏ See therapy plan for specific therapy goals.	_____
❏ Improve function ❏ Lessen complications ❏ Manage pain	_____
	_____
	_____

INTERVENTIONS

NURSING	Other Disciplines
1. See therapist treatment plan treatment.	
2. Prepare and transport to therapy _____.	
Time/Days	
3. Special Nursing Instructions:	
❏ Give pain med _____ min. prior to treatment.	
❏ _____	
❏ _____	
❏ _____	

Respiratory Treatments

❏ IMMEDIATE NEEDS CARE PLAN	❏ CORE CARE PLAN
Respiratory Treatments Seven Days	
CMI: Special Care MDS Item: P1bdA = 7	

Resident Name	Date

PROBLEM/NEED RELATED TO	**RESULTING IN**	**STRENGTHS TO DRAW ON**
❏ History of COPD	❏ Shortness of breath/anxiety	❏ Able to communicate needs
❏ Asthma	❏ _____	❏ Able to follow directions
❏ _____	❏ _____	❏ _____
❏ _____		

GOAL(S)	**TARGET/REVIEW DATE**
❏ Lungs will be clear to auscultation. ❏ Respirations will be unlabored.	
❏ _____	
❏ _____	
❏ _____	

INTERVENTIONS

NURSING	DIETARY
❏ Monitor vital signs: Freq _____.	
❏ Assess lung fields/breath sounds: Freq _____.	
❏ Evaluate shortness of breath for pain/discomfort with breathing.	
❏ Provide PRN medications; cough, pain, discomfort, anxiety.	
❏ Instruct resident in breathing techniques: purse lip, cough and deep breathing: Freq _____.	
❏ Provide oxygen at ____ Liters per min: ___ Intermittent ___ Continuous ___Mask ___ Nasal cannula.	
❏ Prevent irritation/pressure from developing from oxygen tubing by:	**SOCIAL SERVICES**
_____.	
❏ Provide respiratory treatments per MD order:	
___ Inhalers: Freq _____	
___ Other _____	
❏ _____	
❏ _____	
❏ _____	
	ACTIVITIES
Notify physician if: Lung field remains diminished or if sounds are absent in any area; increased complaints of difficulty breathing.	

Seizure Disorder

❑ IMMEDIATE NEEDS CARE PLAN	❑ CORE CARE PLAN
Seizure Disorder	

Resident Name	Date

PROBLEM/NEED RELATED TO	RESULTING IN	STRENGTHS TO DRAW ON
❑ Unknown cause ❑ Anoxia ❑ Brain tumor ❑ CVA ❑ _____	❑ Focal seizures ❑ Generalizes seizures ❑ Status epilepticus ❑ _____	❑ Aware of aura that precedes seizure activity. ❑ Able to communicate needs. ❑ _____

GOAL(S)	TARGET/REVIEW DATE
❑ Resident will be free of seizure activity. ❑ Resident will be protected from harm in the event a seizure occurs. ❑ _____	

INTERVENTIONS

NURSING	DIETARY
❑ Provide medication as ordered. ❑ Monitor for signs/symptoms of toxic effects from medication (e.g., lethargy, dizziness, drowsiness, slurred speech, irritability, nausea/vomiting.) ❑ Monitor lab work as ordered. Report results to MD. ❑ Should seizure occur: 　·　Avoid restraining the resident during the seizure. 　·　Help the resident to a lying position and loosen any tight clothing. 　·　Clear area of hard objects. Place something soft under the head. 　·　**Do not** force anything in the mouth during the seizure. 　·　Keep head turned to maintain open airway. ❑ After seizure: 　·　Reassure resident, orient resident to time and place, inform him/her of having had a seizure. 　·　Assess vital signs. Assist to bed for rest post seizure. 　·　Document length of time, type of seizure, and resident responsiveness. 　·　Notify MD and family. ❑ _____ ❑ _____ ❑ _____	
	SOCIAL SERVICES
	ACTIVITIES

Septicemia

☐ IMMEDIATE NEEDS CARE PLAN	☐ CORE CARE PLAN
Septicemia	
CMI: Clinically Complex	**MDS Item: 12g = checked**

Resident Name	Date

PROBLEM/NEED RELATED TO	RESULTING IN/RISK FOR	STRENGTHS TO DRAW ON
☐ Acute Infection	☐ Fever ☐ Vomiting	☐ _____
☐ Unknown Cause	☐ Dehydration	☐ _____
☐ _____	☐ _____	
☐ _____		

GOAL(S)	TARGET/REVIEW DATE
☐ Will be free of symptoms of infection: Vital signs within normal limits, no drainage.	
☐ Vomiting will be controlled and hydration will be maintained /restored.	
☐ _____	

INTERVENTIONS

NURSING	DIETARY
☐ Monitor vital signs: Freq _____.	☐ Provide diet change until problem resolved.
Monitor for signs of shock.	☐ Check lab: _____ Freq _____.
☐ Monitor lab work as ordered: Culture and sensitivity: Freq _____.	☐ _____
☐ Provide fluid and medications, administration per MD order. See IV POC, IV medications POC.	
☐ Monitor for adverse side effect of ordered antibiotics, if present, stop immediately and notify MD.	**SOCIAL SERVICES**
☐ Utilize universal precautions in providing care.	
☐ Provide IV fluids and medications per MD order: See IV and IV med POC.	
☐ _____	
☐ _____	
Notify physician if: Fever persists; vital signs diminish; cultures are abnormal; drug sensitivities are noted.	**ACTIVITIES**

Skin Breakdown, Risk for

☐ IMMEDIATE NEEDS CARE PLAN	☐ CORE CARE PLAN
Risk for Skin Breakdown	

Resident Name	Date

PROBLEM/NEED RELATED TO	KEY RISK AREA(s)			STRENGTHS TO DRAW ON
☐ Disease/Diagnosis _____	☐ Back of head			☐ Able to cooperate
☐ Cast ☐ Splint	☐ Ears	Left	Right	☐ Drinks fluids liberally
☐ Limited/poor mobility	☐ Elbows	Left	Right	☐ Consumes adequate calories
☐ Inactivity ☐ Sensory Loss	☐ Shoulders	Left	Right	
☐ Inadequate nutrition	☐ Sacrum			
☐ Inadequate hydration	☐ Buttocks			
☐ Fragile skin/poor turgor	☐ Hip(s)	Left	Right	
☐ Incontinence of bowel	☐ Shins	Left	Right	
☐ Incontinence of bladder	☐ Heels	Left	Right	
☐ Resistance to care/non-compliant	☐ Other _____			
☐ _____				

GOAL(S)	TARGET/REVIEW DATE
☐ Skin will remain free of breakdown.	
☐ Reddened areas will be promptly identified and treatment initiated.	
☐ _____	

INTERVENTIONS

NURSING	DIETARY
☐ Complete skin risk assessment weekly x 4, then monthly in conjunction with skin integrity nurse's note.	
☐ Follow ADL Care Directives.	
☐ STNA assess skin condition with daily care. Report results to nurse in charge.	
☐ Total body check with all showers and complete baths.	
☐ If poor or limited mobility turn/redistribute weight every _____ hours.	
☐ Ensure pressure-reducing mattress is in place and functional each day.	**SOCIAL SERVICES**
☐ Use _____ cushion while up in chair.	
☐ Maintain hourly chair positioning schedule, shifting weight. If able, have resident shift weight every 15 minutes. Prompt if needed.	
☐ Prevent skin-to-skin to contact. Use _____ between skin surfaces; ____ use pillows for support ___ use wedge cushions.	
☐ If dependent use two-person assist for turns and positioning.	
☐ Follow continence management plan.	
☐ Protect skin from moisture. Use ___ barrier cream __ soapless cleaner other _____.	**ACTIVITIES**
☐ Record food intake each meal. Report intake less than _____ to nurse.	
☐ Provide and encourage fluids at each meal and in between.	
☐ _____	

Skin Tear

❏ IMMEDIATE NEEDS CARE PLAN	❏ CORE CARE PLAN
Skin Tear	

Resident Name	Date

RESULTING IN	STRENGTHS TO DRAW ON
❏ Arm left right ❏ Leg left right ❏ Other _____ Description of site: _____ _____ _____	

GOAL(S)	TARGET/REVIEW DATE
❏ Skin tear will resolve without complication.	

INTERVENTIONS

NURSING	DIETARY
❏ Check site and change dressing: Freq _____ . ❏ Treatment as ordered. ❏ Observe site for infection, inflammation, redness, and tenderness. ❏ Take extra care during transfer, handling resident. ❏ Continue interventions on at-risk plan in place. ❏ Modify at-risk plan in place. ❏ Develop at-risk plan. ❏ _____ ❏ _____ ❏ _____	
	SOCIAL SERVICES
	ACTIVITIES

Suicidal

☐ IMMEDIATE NEEDS CARE PLAN	☐ CORE CARE PLAN
Suicidal	

Resident Name	Date

PROBLEM/NEED RELATED TO	RESULTING IN	STRENGTHS TO DRAW ON
☐ Major Depression ☐ End-stage disease process ☐ Social isolation, absence of support ☐ Major psychosis ☐ _____	☐ Refusal of medications/treatments ☐ Weight loss ☐ Refusal to eat ☐ Feelings of hopelessness/helplessness ☐ Suicidal thoughts or attempts (describe): _____	☐ Will express feelings ☐ Able to understand ☐ Responds to redirection ☐ _____ ☐ _____

GOAL(S)	TARGET/REVIEW DATE
☐ Resident will not harm self. ☐ Depression will be lifted and thoughts of suicide will dissipate. ☐ _____ ☐ _____	

INTERVENTIONS

NURSING

☐ Monitor resident's whereabouts and activities: Freq _____.
☐ Institute safety precautions for suicide risk:

_____

_____.

☐ Monitor and document suicidal ideation, response to interventions and use of medications. Discuss status with physician: Freq _____.
☐ Encourage verbalization of feelings. Use reflective questioning technique (e.g., "You feel your life is over?").
☐ Allow choices where it will not create harm.
☐ _____
☐ _____
☐ _____
☐ _____

Should an attempt be made: Assess for medical needs, notify the MD and family. Provide emergency interventions as indicated.

DIETARY

☐ Provide meals with paper/plastic products as indicated.
☐ Liberalize diet to items resident will eat
☐ _____

SOCIAL SERVICES

☐ Counseling daily, allow to process feelings. Document response/progress each visit.
☐ Facilitate professional counseling with psychologist/psychiatrist.
☐ _____
☐ _____
☐ _____

ACTIVITIES

☐ Involve in structured activities as able.
☐ Provide divisional activity:
Type: _____

_____
Freq: _____
Instruction for nursing staff:

Surgical Wound with Treatment

❑ IMMEDIATE NEEDS CARE PLAN	❑ CORE CARE PLAN
Surgical Wound with Treatment	
CMI: Special Care MDS Item: M4g and M5f = Checked	

Resident Name	Date

PROBLEM/NEED RELATED TO	RESULTING IN	STRENGTHS TO DRAW ON
❑ Hip repair	❑ Surgical wound location:	❑ Able to communicate needs
❑ Abdominal surgery: Specify	_____	❑ Able to follow directions
	_____	❑ _____
_____		
❑ Amputation	❑ _____	❑ _____
❑ _____		

GOAL(S)	TARGET/REVIEW DATE
❑ Surgical wound will be healed without complication.	
❑ _____	
❑ _____	

INTERVENTIONS

NURSING	DIETARY
❑ Monitor vital signs: Freq _____.	❑ Increase protein needs: Provide supplements as ordered to promote healing:_____.
❑ Wound status: Approximation of wound, assessment of surrounding tissue, presence of staples, sutures where applicable.	❑ Recommend vitamins for wound healing.
❑ Complaints of pain, effectiveness of pain medication per MD order.	❑ Check lab: _____ Freq _____
❑ Apply medicated ointment per MD order.	❑ Evaluate weights: Freq _____.
❑ Apply dressing per MD order: _____.	❑ _____
_____	**SOCIAL SERVICES**
❑ Note old dressing for any signs of exudate. Assess color and amount if present.	
❑ Be alert to any signs of infection: drainage, odor, redness of surrounding tissue, red streaking up the extremity.	
❑ Remove sutures/staples per MD order: _____	
_____	
❑ Follow up appointment: _____	
❑ Keep dietary informed of wound status: Freq _____.	
❑ _____	**ACTIVITIES**
❑ _____	
❑ _____	
Notify physician if: Wound status unchanged for two weeks in row; evidence of change in or deterioration in status of wound; symptoms of infection.	

Trach/Suctioning

☐ IMMEDIATE NEEDS CARE PLAN	☐ CORE CARE PLAN
Tracheotomy/Suctioning	
CMI: Extensive Services MDS Item: P1i and P1j	

Resident Name	Date

PROBLEM/NEED RELATED TO	RESULTING IN	STRENGTHS TO DRAW ON
☐ History of COPD	☐ Cough: non-productive	☐ Able to communicate needs.
☐ _____	☐ Cough: productive	☐ Able to follow instruction.
☐ _____	☐ Unable to clear secretions, suctioning required	☐ _____
☐ _____	☐ Shortness of breath	☐ _____
	☐ Anxiety	☐ _____
	☐ _____	

GOAL(S)	TARGET/REVIEW DATE
☐ Breathing will be non-labored.	
☐ Trach will be patent, free of occlusion.	
☐ Anxiety will be controlled with use of _____.	
☐ _____	

INTERVENTIONS

NURSING	DIETARY
☐ Monitor vital signs: Freq _____.	
☐ Assess lung fields/breath sounds: Freq _____.	
☐ Evaluate shortness of breath for pain/discomfort, anxiety, fluid in lungs.	
☐ Evaluate and document sputum/increased secretions.	
☐ Suction PRN as ordered. Record frequency/number of times each shift.	
☐ Provide trach care as ordered and PRN for increased secretions.	
☐ Minimize irritation of trach site by _____.	
☐ Give antibiotics as ordered, monitoring drug adverse reactions/side effects.	**SOCIAL SERVICES**
☐ Give PRN meds as indicated for cough, pain/discomfort, anxiety.	
☐ Allay fears, instruct as to what you are doing, provide reassurance.	
☐ Refer also to Respiratory Therapy plan.	
☐ _____	
☐ _____	
Notify physician if: Adverse reaction from medications, sputum changes in color, consistency, amount indicating worsening, diminished or absent lung sounds, increasing complaints of shortness of breath and escalating/ uncontrolled anxiety.	**ACTIVITIES**

❏ IMMEDIATE NEEDS CARE PLAN	❏ CORE CARE PLAN
Transfusion	
CMI: Clinically Complex	**MDS Item: P1k = checked**

Resident Name	Date

PROBLEM/NEED RELATED TO	**RESULTING IN/RISK FOR**	**STRENGTHS TO DRAW ON**
❏ Internal bleed	❏ Postural hypotension, tachycardia	❏ _____
❏ Trauma	❏ Fatigue, shortness of breath, pallor, rapid thready pulse	❏ _____
❏ Anemia	❏ _____	
❏ Chemotherapy side effects	❏ _____	
❏ _____		
❏ _____		

GOAL(S)	**TARGET/REVIEW DATE**
❏ Free of transfusion reaction. ❏ No complaints of fatigue, shortness or breath.	
❏ _____	

INTERVENTIONS

NURSING	DIETARY
❏ Evaluate IV site to assure no signs of infiltrate: redness or complaints of pain at site. If present, restart IV site prior to initiation of blood transfusion.	
❏ Administration set up with filter and Y-tubing: connected to 250 – 500 cc bag of normal saline for infusion.	
❏ Double-check blood type and blood unit information with second nurse prior to hanging any blood product.	
❏ Vital signs prior to administration as baseline, fifteen minutes after initiation of infusion and then (Freq) _____ until blood transfusion completed.	
❏ Provide pre-medication per MD orders: _____.	**SOCIAL SERVICES**
❏ Stay with resident first fifteen minutes of infusion and observe any adverse reaction (e.g., increased respiration, rash or hive-like eruptions). If present, stop infusion, change tubing, and run normal saline; notify MD immediately. Provide emergency measures per MD order:	
_____;	
Notify the lab of possible blood reaction.	
❏ Regulate flow to infuse packed cells within ____ hrs. Whole blood within ____ hrs.	**ACTIVITIES**
❏ If other medication or fluids to be provided, use second IV site. See IV POC.	
❏ Assess follow up lab work per MD order: Hg and HCT Freq _____.	
❏ _____	
Notify physician if: Symptoms of blood reaction; symptoms of bleed identified; abnormal lab work; bleeding persists; vital signs diminish.	

Tube Feed 51% or More

❏ IMMEDIATE NEEDS CARE PLAN   ❏ CORE CARE PLAN
Tube Feed 51% or 26% Calories and 501+ cc/day fluid
CMI: Clinically complex   MDS Item: K5b and/or K6a = 2 and K6b = 2, 3, 4   QI: Tube Feed

OR

Tube Feed: With Fever: 51% Calories or 26% Calories and 501cc fluid per day last seven days
CMI: Special Care   MDS Item: K5b and J1k, K5B and K6a = 2, 3, 4   QI: Tube Feed

Resident Name	Date

PROBLEM/NEED RELATED TO	RESULTING IN	STRENGTHS TO DRAW ON
❏ Chewing problem	❏ Fever	❏ Able to communicate needs
❏ Swallowing problem	❏ Risk of aspiration	❏ Able to follow directions
❏ Dysphagia ❏ Resisting eating	❏ Risk of infection at insertion site	❏ _____
❏ Weight Loss ❏ Coma	❏ _____	❏ _____
❏ Depression	❏ _____	
❏ _____		

GOAL(S)	TARGET/REVIEW DATE
❏ Will be free of aspiration. ❏ Insertion site will be free of symptoms of infection.	
❏ Will maintain current weight of ____ +/- ____ lbs.	
❏ Will have oral intake of _____% each meal.	
❏ _____	

INTERVENTIONS

NURSING

❏ Placement of tube by aspiration and osculation: Hold feed if greater than _____ cc aspirate.
❏ Listen to lung sounds: Freq _____.
❏ Vital signs: Freq _____ Assess source of fever: Rule out UTI, infected insertion site, lung infection.
❏ Monitor side effects: diarrhea, nausea/vomiting, increased cough or shortness of breath.
❏ Describe actual amounts of tube feed formula received each shift and water received each shift.
❏ Monitor insertion site of tube for symptoms of infection.
❏ Keep HOB elevated 45 degrees during and thirty minutes after tube feed.
❏ Administer tube feed: Type _____ Amount _____ Frequency _____.
❏ Control volume delivered using TF pump.
❏ Administer medication as ordered.
❏ Document TF and water intake QS.
❏ _____

Notify physician if: Symptoms of diarrhea, nausea/vomiting; held tube feed, calorie or fluid need changes; lung field remains diminished or if sounds are absent in any area; increased complaints of difficulty breathing; abnormal lab; persistent fever.

DIETARY

❏ Nursing to alert if fluid intake compromised.
❏ Provide supplements as ordered: _____.
❏ Check lab: _____ Freq _____.
❏ Assure fluid intake to ___ ccs q 24 hrs.
❏ If combined with oral feed: Plug or clamp tube feed for time/freq _____.
❏ Evaluate oral feedings compared to need for TF: Freq _____.
❏ _____

SOCIAL SERVICES

ACTIVITIES

Tube Feed with Aphasia

❏ IMMEDIATE NEEDS CARE PLAN   ❏ CORE CARE PLAN

Tube Feed with Aphasia

CMI: Special Care   MDS Item: K5b and I1r   QI: Tube Feed

Resident Name	Date

PROBLEM/NEED RELATED TO	RESULTING IN	STRENGTHS TO DRAW ON
❏ Chewing problem ❏ Swallowing problem ❏ Dysphagia ❏ Resisting eating ❏ Weight Loss ❏ Depression ❏ _____	❏ Risk of aspiration ❏ Inability to express distress ❏ _____ ❏ _____	❏ Able to follow directions ❏ _____ ❏ _____

GOAL(S)	TARGET/REVIEW DATE
❏ Will be free of aspiration. ❏ Will maintain current weight of ____ +/- ____ lbs. ❏ Will have oral intake of _____% each meal. ❏ Will communicate needs with use of _____. ❏ _____	

INTERVENTIONS

NURSING

❏ Placement of tube by aspiration and osculation: Hold feed if greater than _____cc aspirate.

❏ Listen to lung sounds: Freq _____.

❏ Vital signs: Freq _____.

❏ Monitor side effects: diarrhea, nausea/vomiting, increased cough or shortness of breath.

❏ Describe actual amounts of tube feed formula received each shift and water received each shift.

❏ Place resident closer to nursing station/view to monitor for signs of distress, increase monitoring of resident status to (Freq) _____.

❏ Monitor insertion site of tube for symptoms of infection.

❏ Keep HOB elevated 45 degrees during and thirty minutes after tube feed.

❏ Administer tube feed: Type _____ Amount _____ Frequency _____. Control volume delivered using TF pump.

❏ _____

❏ _____

Notify physician if: Symptoms of diarrhea, nausea/vomiting; held tube feed, calorie or fluid need changes; lung field remains diminished or if sounds are absent in any area; increased complaints of difficulty breathing; abnormal lab.

DIETARY

❏ Nursing to alert if fluid intake compromised.

❏ Provide supplements as ordered: _____.

❏ Check lab: _____ Freq _____.

❏ Assure fluid intake to ___ ccs q 24 hrs.

❏ If combined with oral feed: Plug or clamp tube feed for time/freq _____.

❏ Evaluate oral feedings compared to need for TF: Freq _____.

❏ _____

SOCIAL SERVICES

ACTIVITIES

Upper Respiratory Infection

❑ IMMEDIATE NEEDS CARE PLAN   ❑ CORE CARE PLAN
Upper Respiratory Infection

Resident Name	Date

RESULTING IN		STRENGTHS TO DRAW ON
❑ Non productive cough ❑ Productive cough		❑ Able to communicate needs
❑ Shortness of breath ❑ Risk for dehydration		❑ Able to follow directions
		❑ Takes fluids liberally
❑ _____		❑ _____
❑ _____		❑ _____
		❑ _____

GOAL(S)	REVIEW DATE
❑ URI will resolve without complications.	
❑ Will consume adequate fluids to prevent dehydration.	
❑ _____	
❑ _____	

INTERVENTIONS

NURSING	DIETARY
❑ Monitor vital signs: Freq _____.	❑ Instruct nursing to alert to compromised fluid intake.
❑ Assess breath sounds: Freq _____.	❑ Assure fluid intake to _____ ccs q hr.
❑ Evaluate shortness of breath for pain/discomfort with breathing, provide meds as ordered.	
❑ Provide extra fluids to keep secretions thin between meals and at bedtime.	
❑ Administer antibiotics. Monitor for any adverse reaction to drug.	
❑ Provide PRN medications for cough, pain, discomfort, anxiety, difficulty resting.	**SOCIAL SERVICES**
❑ Refer to Respiratory Therapy.	
❑ _____	
❑ _____	
❑ _____	
❑ _____	
Notify physician if: Any adverse reaction to antibiotic: stop medication, note reaction symptoms; sputum changes in color; lung field unusual (rales, etc.); increased complaints of difficulty breathing, persistent fever.	**ACTIVITIES**

Urinary Incontinence

❑ IMMEDIATE NEEDS CARE PLAN	❑ CORE CARE PLAN
Urinary Incontinence	

Resident Name	Date

Type of Incontinence	**STRENGTHS TO DRAW ON**
❑ Functional: ❑ physical ❑ mental ❑ both	❑ Aware of urge to void
❑ Urge Incontinence (abrupt loss of urine)	❑ Yes ❑ No ❑ Occ.
❑ Overflow Incontinence (constant dribble)	❑ Can cooperate with toileting
❑ Stress Incontinence (spurts of urine)	❑ Yes ❑ No ❑ Occ.
❑ Obstruction or stricture	❑ Mobility status
❑ Unable to determine	❑ Indep. ❑ Supervise ❑ Assist
❑ Other _____	❑ Dependent
	❑ Able to manage clothing
	❑ Yes ❑ No
	❑ Able to wipe self
	❑ Yes ❑ No

GOAL(S)	**TARGET/REVIEW DATE**
❑ Dependent Continence: continent thru efforts of others.	
❑ Social Continence: clean, dry, odor free.	
❑ Incontinent episodes < 1x/w : usually will be continent.	
❑ 2 or >/wk but not daily: only occasionally incontinent.	

INTERVENTIONS

NURSING	DIETARY
❑ **Habit training**: no pattern established.	
Toilet every _____(days/eves/nites). Clean and change if needed.	
❑ **Scheduled** based on voiding pattern established.	
Toilet every _____(days/eves/nites). Clean and change if needed.	
❑ **Prompted**: occ./always aware of need; has voiding pattern.	SOCIAL SERVICES
Toilet every _____ (days/eves/nites). Clean and change if needed.	
Check and change/P&P.	
❑ Bladder Retraining Protocol.	
❑ **See restorative program for** _____.	ACTIVITIES
❑ _____	
❑ _____	

Urinary Tract Infection

☐ IMMEDIATE NEEDS CARE PLAN	☐ CORE CARE PLAN
Urinary Tract Infection ☐ Risk for ☐ Active Infection ☐ Chronic Infection	

Resident Name	Date

PROBLEM/NEED RELATED TO	STRENGTHS TO DRAW ON
☐ History of UTI creating further risk ☐ Presence of catheter ☐ Poor toileting habits ☐ Poor fluid intake ☐ Active infection with sx of UTI (urgency, frequency, pain, fever, abnormal labs) ☐ Chronic asymptomatic Infection ☐ _____	☐ Readily drinks fluids ☐ Able to communicate needs ☐ Able to follow directions ☐ _____ ☐ _____

GOAL(S)	TARGET/REVIEW DATE
☐ Will be free of signs and symptoms of UTI.	
☐ Catheter will be discontinued by _____ and resident will void without difficulty.	
☐ Urine will be clear and light-colored without heavy sediment.	
☐ _____	

INTERVENTIONS

NURSING	DIETARY
☐ Assess urinary status (freq) _____ evaluating color, odor, amount. ☐ Provide fluids to flush urinary system: 1500-2000 cc daily unless contraindicated. ☐ Encourage fluids between meals and with medication administration. ☐ Monitor TPR and BP Freq: _____. ☐ Instruct resident to void as soon as urge is felt. ☐ Toilet per plan. ☐ Provide/assist/instruct on proper peri-care. ☐ Provide pain and antipyretic medication per MD orders. Document effectiveness. ☐ Catheter care per policy. ☐ Labs as ordered. ☐ _____ ☐ _____ ☐ _____	☐ Provide cranberry juice with each meal. ☐ _____ ☐ _____ ☐ _____
	SOCIAL SERVICES
	ACTIVITIES
Notify physician if: Symptoms continue past treatment orders; pain persists; lab work positive.	☐ Provide fluids during activities attended. ☐ Encourage attendance at activities involving snacks and drinks.

Vent/Trach/Suctioning

❑ IMMEDIATE NEEDS CARE PLAN	❑ CORE CARE PLAN
Tracheotomy/Suctioning/Ventilator Support	
CMI: Extensive Services MDS Item: P1i and P1j and P1L	

Resident Name	Date

PROBLEM/NEED RELATED TO	RESULTING IN	STRENGTHS TO DRAW ON
❑ History of COPD	❑ Inability to clear secretions	❑ Able to communicate needs.
❑ Coma	❑ Continuous ventilator support	❑ Able to follow instruction.
❑ _____	❑ Intermittent ventilator support	❑ _____
❑ _____	❑ _____	❑ _____

GOAL(S)	TARGET/REVIEW DATE
❑ Respirations will be easy, unlabored.	
❑ Trach will be patent, free of occlusion.	
❑ _____	
❑ _____	

INTERVENTIONS

NURSING	DIETARY
❑ Monitor vital signs: Freq _____.	
❑ Assess lung fields/breath sounds: Freq _____.	
❑ Evaluate shortness of breath for pain/discomfort, anxiety, fluid in lungs.	
❑ Evaluate and document sputum/increased secretions.	
❑ Suction PRN as ordered. Record frequency/number of times each shift.	
❑ Provide trach care as ordered and PRN for increased secretions.	
❑ Minimize irritation of trach site by _____.	
❑ Ventilator settings/MD order.	**SOCIAL SERVICES**
❑ Respond promptly to alarm sounding. Evaluate cause and correct. If unable to correct, ambu bag resident, attempt to suction.	
❑ Give antibiotics as ordered monitoring drug adverse reactions/side effects.	
❑ Give PRN meds as indicated for cough, pain/discomfort, anxiety.	
❑ Allay fears, instruct as to what you are doing, provide reassurance.	
❑ Refer also to Respiratory Therapy plan.	
❑ _____	
❑ _____	
Notify physician if: Adverse reaction from medications, sputum changes in color, consistency, amount indicating worsening, diminished or absent lung sounds, airway difficulties not relieved by suctioning.	**ACTIVITIES**

The Big Book of Care Plans, Second Edition

Weight Gain, Unplanned

❑ IMMEDIATE NEEDS CARE PLAN	❑ CORE CARE PLAN
Unplanned/Unexpected Weight Gain	

Resident Name	Date

PROBLEM/NEED RELATED TO	RESULTING IN/RISK FOR	STRENGTHS TO DRAW ON
❑ Cardiac disease	❑ Peripheral edema ❑ UE ❑ LE	❑ Alert and able to communicate hunger
❑ Diuretic use	❑ Pulmonary edema	❑ Complies with medical regimen
❑ Overeating	❑ Difficulty determining nutrition	❑ _____
❑ _____	status	❑ _____
❑ _____	❑ Difficulty controlling blood sugars	❑ _____
❑ _____	❑ _____	❑ _____

GOAL(S)	TARGET/REVIEW DATE
❑ Weight will range between _____ and _____ lbs. ❑ daily ❑ weekly ❑ monthly.	
❑ Will not develop pulmonary edema.	
❑ Will consume ____50% ____75% ___100% two of three meals/day.	
❑ Nutrition will be adequate as evidenced by _____.	
❑ _____	

INTERVENTIONS

NURSING	DIETARY
Provide mealtime assist/ADL directives.	Check weight status at least _____.
❑ Weigh at same time of day and record: Freq _____.	Determine nutritional adequacy based on
❑ Monitor and record food intake at each meal.	_____.
❑ If weight is not within range, contact physician.	
❑ Give supplements as ordered. Alert dietitian if not consuming on a routine basis.	
❑ Report ordered lab results to physician; ensure dietitian is aware.	
❑ _____	
❑ _____	SOCIAL SERVICES
❑ _____	
❑ _____	
❑ _____	
❑ _____	
Notify MD if: Increasing shortness of breath; escalating edema; increased anxiety; inability to lie flat; change in baseline level of orientation/alertness.	ACTIVITIES

Weight Loss, Unplanned

❏ IMMEDIATE NEEDS CARE PLAN	❏ CORE CARE PLAN
Unplanned/Unexpected Weight Loss	

Resident Name	Date

PROBLEM/NEED RELATED TO	RESULTING IN RISK FOR	STRENGTHS TO DRAW ON
❏ Recent hospitalization	❏ Malnutrition	❏ Alert and able to communicate hunger
❏ Acute illness	❏ _____	❏ Appetite returning to baseline
❏ Poor food intake	❏ _____	❏ _____
❏ _____		❏ _____

GOAL(S)	TARGET/REVIEW DATE
Weight will return to baseline range between _____ and _____ lbs.	
Will regain weight at _____ lbs. per month.	
Will consume ____50% ____75% ___100% two of three meals/day.	
❏ _____	

INTERVENTIONS

NURSING	DIETARY
❏ Monitor and record food intake at each meal.	
❏ Offer substitutes as requested or indicated.	
❏ Alert dietitian if consumption is poor more than 48 hours.	
❏ Weigh at same time of day and record: Freq _____.	
❏ If weight decline persists, contact physician and dietitian immediately.	
❏ Give supplements as ordered. Alert dietitian if not consuming on a routine basis.	
❏ Labs as ordered. Report results to physician and ensure dietician is aware.	**SOCIAL SERVICES**
❏ Refer to ADL directives for specifics of care to be provided.	
❏ Refer to restorative feeding program POC.	
❏ _____	
❏ _____	
❏ _____	
❏ _____	**ACTIVITIES**

The Big Book of Care Plans, Second Edition

Weight Loss with Fever

❑ IMMEDIATE NEEDS CARE PLAN	❑ CORE CARE PLAN
Fever with Weight Loss	
CMI: Special Care	**MDS Item: J1h and J1a = checked or K3a = 1**

Resident Name	Date

PROBLEM/NEED RELATED TO	RESULTING IN	STRENGTHS TO DRAW ON
❑ Acute infection	❑ Temperature above 100 degrees rectal	❑ Able to communicate needs
❑ Flu	❑ Emesis ❑ Weakness	❑ Able to follow directions
❑ Bowel obstruction	❑ Risk for dehydration	❑ _____
❑ Psychogenic	❑ Weight loss 3 lbs. last seven days or last	❑ _____
❑ Chemotherapy	30 days	
❑ Radiation Therapy	❑ _____	
❑ Unknown cause	❑ _____	
❑ _____		

GOAL(S)	TARGET/REVIEW DATE
❑ Fever and vomiting will resolve without complication.	
❑ Free of symptoms of dehydration as evidenced by moist mucous membranes, good skin turgor.	
❑ Will eat 75 – 100 % of meals ❑ Will stabilize weight between ____ lbs. and ___ lbs.	
❑ _____	

INTERVENTIONS

NURSING	DIETARY
❑ Vital signs: Freq _____.	❑ Provide high-calorie, high-fat products on trays unless contraindicated.
❑ Weight: Freq _____. Notify dietitian if weight loss continues.	❑ Provide supplements as ordered:
❑ Bowel sounds, frequency of BM, type and amount of BM daily.	_____.
❑ Signs of dehydration: tenting skin, dry mouth, cracked lips, dizziness on sitting/standing, fever, increased pulse, thirst, weakness, weight loss.	❑ Check lab: _____ Freq _____.
❑ Lab work: BUN creatinine electrolytes as ordered.	❑ Evaluate weights: Freq _____
❑ Assess urine output for symptoms of dehydration: concentrated urine, strong odor.	❑ _____
❑ Provide antipyretic, antiemetic medication per MD orders.	**SOCIAL SERVICES**
❑ If related to recent chemotherapy, provide bland, soft foods. Avoid spicy foods.	
❑ Provide foods of choice: _____.	
❑ _____	
❑ _____	
❑ _____	**ACTIVITIES**
❑ _____	
Notify physician if: Persistent weight loss; abnormal lab; persistent fever above 100 degrees rectal.	